I0091015

The creative process is _____

Ritual

Ritual is the means whereby the individual is able to position or align the self in such a way that the creative process delivers to the individual a specific desired outcome, effortlessly, as if from an outside source.

Bindling

Bindling is a ritual wherein the individual effortlessly releases excess weight and permanently maintains desired bodily form by focusing simply on deliberately creating the powerful psychospiritual condition of self-mastery—and thereby turning over the task of releasing excess weight and permanently maintaining desired bodily form to the creative process as it is manifested in the deeper levels of the psyche.

Bindling is a technique of ecstasy, which produces multiple levels of ecstasy that reinforce and energize the ongoing bindling process.

In the ritual of bindling, the individual creates the powerful psychospiritual condition of self-mastery by creating a repeated daily pattern of (a) obtaining and documenting food to be eaten one day in advance and (b) following through with this plan on the designated day.

When the individual creates the condition of self-mastery in this way, this initiates the activation of a deep, underlying psychospiritual process whereby the individual's desired bodily form becomes delivered to the individual by the creative process.

This Book

This book is a comprehensive guide to the ritual of bindling and to the underlying psychospiritual process that the bindling ritual activates. The book is divided into two main sections (see directory on back cover); the first main section is (a) the bindling concept section (note that we are in the bindling concept section right now), and the second main section is (b) the bindling process section.

Bindling Concept

The ritual of bindling revolves around the concept of the paradox of effortlessness. In the bindling concept section, we explore the paradox of effortlessness as it relates to the ritual of bindling, and we examine the various interrelated concepts that revolve around this basic, core concept.

Bindling Process

The bindling process section includes specific, detailed instructions regarding how to participate in the ritual of bindling. These specific instructions appear in the chapter on How to Bindle.

The bindling process section also includes a series of chapters that describe the deeper, underlying psychospiritual process that is activated through participation in the ritual of bindling (see chapters on Self-Mastery, Transformation of Self, Condition of Inevitability, and Desired Outcome).

These chapters on the deeper psychospiritual process that is activated through the ritual of bindling include specific guidance regarding how to stay out of the way of the creative process while it does its work (see chapter on Transformation of Self). These chapters also include specific guidance regarding how to gently accelerate the momentum of the process such that the individual's desired bodily form becomes materialized as quickly and as effectively as is possible (see chapter on Condition of Inevitability).

The book concludes with a chapter in which the individual is guided through a Three-Day Initiation Cycle, wherein the individual initiates the bindling process and thereby enters into the powerful psychospiritual condition of self-mastery.

Forms that are used for the Three-Day Initiation Cycle and 100 days of bindling are provided at the end of the Three-Day Initiation Cycle chapter.

Bindling – In Summary

Bindling is a ritual wherein the individual focuses simply on deliberately creating the powerful psychospiritual condition of self-mastery in as effortless a manner as is possible, and thereby turns over the task of releasing excess weight and permanently maintaining desired bodily form to the creative process as it is manifested in the deeper levels of the psyche.

In the ritual of bindling, the individual creates the powerful psychospiritual condition of self-mastery by creating a repeated daily pattern of (a) obtaining and documenting food to be eaten one day in advance and (b) following through with this plan on the designated day.

Bindling is a simple, few-minutes-daily ritual that is fully amenable to the unique contours of the life of the individual. For example, bindling allows for full participation in social eating rituals and other important eating occasions.

The ritual of bindling is described in full detail in the How to Bindle chapter. Before we get to that though, let's have a look at the basic concept around which the ritual of bindling revolves — the basic concept of the paradox of effortlessness.

Dieting as an Art Form

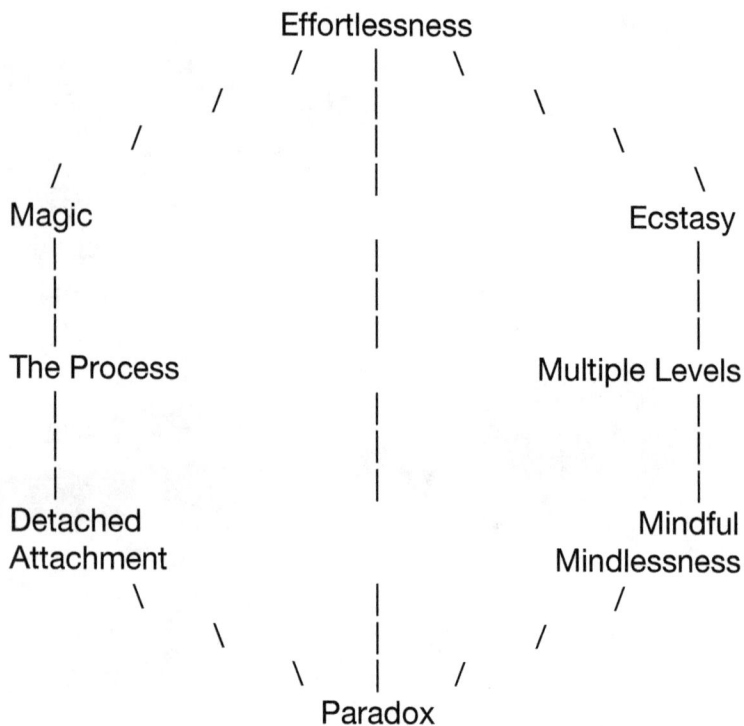

Effortlessness
/ | \
/ | \
/ | \
/ | \
Magic Ecstasy
|
|
|
The Process Multiple Levels
|
|
|
Detached Mindful
Attachment Mindlessness
\ | /
\ | /
\ | /
Paradox

Effortlessness

Our initial experiences of food occur within the effortless space of the womb. In the ritual of bindling, the individual recreates the effortless space of the womb in a manner that is conducive with the individual's desired bodily form.

In the ritual of bindling, effortlessness is achieved by means of magic and ecstasy.

Effortlessness: Magic

The magic aspect of the effortlessness of the bindling ritual is manifested in the individual simply creating the powerful psychospiritual condition of self-mastery, and thereby turning over the task of releasing excess weight and permanently maintaining desired bodily form to the creative process as it is manifested in the deeper levels of the psyche.

The real work of releasing excess weight and permanently maintaining desired bodily form is carried out not by the individual, but by the creative process. Bindling is merely the gesture, the ritual gesture that sets this process into motion.

The introduction of unnecessary effort into this process by the individual blocks the creative process from delivering the desired outcome as quickly and as effectively as is possible.

Bindling is a technique that keeps the individual out of the way of the creative process, so that the creative process can do its work.

Turning over the task of releasing excess weight and permanently maintaining desired bodily form to the creative process is an act of trust.

After the individual turns this task over to the creative process, that is when the real magic occurs. The creative process then comes up with surprising ways to deliver the desired outcome to the individual as quickly and as effectively as is possible.

By participation in this act of magic, the individual achieves complete freedom from ever again having to be concerned about the task of releasing excess weight and permanently maintaining desired bodily form. This desired outcome becomes automatically programmed into the life of the individual.

Energy that was formerly wrapped up in concern over this specific desired outcome becomes freed up, and the individual then becomes able to channelize this newfound energy into the fulfillment of the individual's life potential.

Effortlessness: Magic – How the Process Works

In the ritual of bindling, the individual focuses simply on creating the powerful psychospiritual condition of self-mastery via the bindling ritual. Meanwhile, within the deeper levels of the psyche, a process is activated whereby the desired outcome is delivered to the individual by the creative process.

This deeper, internal process operates as follows:

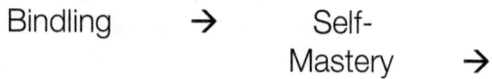

Bindling → Self-Mastery →

Transformation
of Self → Condition of
Inevitability → Desired
Outcome

Through the ritual of <u>bindling</u>, the individual enters into the powerful psychospiritual condition of <u>self-mastery</u>. By entering into the condition of self-mastery in this way, the individual initiates the activation of a deep, underlying <u>transformation of self</u> process. In the transformation of self process, the creative process carries out a comprehensive transformation of the psyche and the life of the individual.

While the creative process carries out the transformation of self, the only task of the individual is to continue to bindle in as effortless a manner as is possible and to stay out of the way of the creative process as it completes the work of transformation.

The individual stays out of the way of the creative process as it completes the work of transformation by dwelling entirely in ecstasy and desire, i.e., by dwelling entirely in (a) the ecstasy that is generated by the ongoing bindling process and in (b) the individual's desire for the outcome. By dwelling entirely in ecstasy and desire in this way, the individual protects the sacred space created by the condition of self-mastery and fully facilitates the transformation of self process.

As the individual continues to bindle and to dwell entirely in ecstasy and desire, the individual enters into the condition of inevitability, which is the condition in which the desired outcome becomes inevitable and materializes.

In the ritual of bindling, effortlessness is achieved by means of magic and ecstasy.

Effortlessness: Ecstasy

The ecstasy aspect of the effortlessness of the bindling ritual is manifested in the ecstasy that the bindling ritual generates. This ecstasy that is generated by the bindling ritual serves to reinforce and energize the ongoing bindling process.

Ecstasy is an innate manifestation of the creative process within the individual. Ecstasy itself is neither good nor bad; rather, it is simply a resource that is available to the individual, which the individual may channelize for the purpose of receiving specific desired outcomes from the creative process.

Actions that are ecstatic feel as if they are happening on their own. They require no pushing or pulling of the self. An ecstatic action is truly effortless.

Bindling operates in full cooperation with the creative process as it is manifested within the individual in the innate flowing processes of desire, pleasure, and ecstasy.

Bindling is not at all about self-denial. Bindling is a technique of ecstasy, and as such it is completely about self-indulgence, and the deepening of ecstasy via paradox.

In fact, it is this deepening of ecstasy that is facilitated by the bindling ritual that facilitates the desired outcome being delivered to the individual as quickly and as effectively as is possible.

Effortlessness: Ecstasy – Multiple Levels

The ritual of bindling generates multiple levels of ecstasy that reinforce and energize the ongoing bindling process.

These multiple levels of process-reinforcing ecstasy are as follows:

The ecstasy of eating
The ecstasy of anticipation
The ecstasy of the process
The ecstasy of self-mastery
The ecstasy of the outcome
The ecstasy of the ripple effects of self-mastery
The ecstasy of containment
The ecstasy of altered consciousness
The ecstasy of freedom

The ecstasy of eating

Eating is the most basic ecstasy. Eating is the ecstasy of survival, the ecstasy of the womb. It is the ecstasy of being surrounded within a warm, nurturing space in which food is effortlessly received into the body.

The ecstasy of receiving food into the body is the most basic ecstasy in the bindling process.

Bindling is a process wherein the individual is able to clear the sensory slate in such a way that the specific foods that are received into the body are experienced with a deeper, more florid sensorial awareness.

This clearing of the sensory slate occurs both due to the basic nature of bindling, in which willy nilly eating is replaced with a more deliberate food selection process, and, on a deeper level, as a result of the participant in bindling being freed up from concern about the release of excess weight and the permanent maintenance of desired bodily form. The desired outcome gets turned over entirely to the creative process, such that the individual becomes available to be entirely present for the ecstatic enjoyment of eating.

The individual who bindles enters into an altered state of consciousness and begins to explore the inner landscapes of various foods in a more direct and intimate manner. Foods that were once thought of as too healthy begin to be experienced in a whole new way, and the hidden ecstasy potential of various foods begins to be discovered. These newfound discoveries occur not on account of any pushing or pulling of the self; rather, they emerge from the innate flowing processes of ecstasy and desire.

Bindling focuses the attention of the individual on the foods that are actually being craved deep down inside. It short circuits willy nilly, impulsive eating and clears the mind in preparation for deeper and more gratifying eating experiences.

Bindling helps the psyche to fully metabolize the experience of being satisfied and satiated by food. The individual who bindles eats in a more mindful, sensual, noticing way, which helps the psyche to realize that it has been satisfied and satiated by the eating process. This fuller metabolizing of satisfaction and satiation plays a key role in the effortless releasing of excess weight and the permanent maintenance of desired bodily form.

Bindling reprograms the mind by deepening its appreciation of both the everyday pleasures of eating and the special occasional novelty of a highly anticipated treat. This reprogramming of the mind has a domino effect in enhancing all of life's pleasures, including both the subtle everyday pleasures and the occasional extraordinary ones, and in deepening the individual's engagement with the very process of life itself.

The ecstasy of anticipation

The individual who bindles always has something to look forward to. The individual who bindles experiences the ecstasy of anticipation both for daily food items and for the individual's desired bodily form, which is delivered to the individual by the creative process.

Also, the individual who bindles experiences the ecstasy of anticipation for the numerous transformations that begin to occur within the psyche and in the life of the individual as a function of the underlying psychospiritual process that is activated by the bindling ritual.

The experience of having something to look forward to is one of the best feelings one can ever have. Oftentimes it is even more satisfying than the actual anticipated event.

The deliberate invocation of the condition of anticipation creates within the self a deep, hollow, magical presence. It colors in all of life's more mundane moments with a mild thrill.

Anticipation is a specific instance of the more general psychospiritual condition of hope. Therefore, the individual who bindles deliberately invokes the psychospiritual condition of hope, and as a result of this, the overall level of hope experienced in the life of the individual begins to increase.

The ecstasy of the process

The ritual of bindling is a creative process, and as such, it is innately rewarding in and of itself.

Creativity is choice, and the individual who bindles gets to experience the daily creative pleasure of making a daily executive decision about what to eat the following day.

The mere act of going through the motions of this daily decision-making process is enjoyable, in and of itself.

Over time, as the bindling process evolves, the individual gets to have the experience of becoming caught up in a valued creative process, and of developing a creative vision for the self. This development of a creative vision is one of the most sublime and powerful of all human experiences. It reverberates throughout the psyche and absorbs the psyche's energy and attention. This in itself can reduce or remove many of a person's cravings for excess food.

The ecstasy of self-mastery

The individual who deliberately creates the condition of self-mastery experiences a sense of accomplishment, confidence, gravitas, a sense of efficacy, personal empowerment, hope, excitement, a sense of adventure, and a feeling of well-being. Self-mastery is championship of the self, and it brings a feeling of inner strength, of being fully alive, and of being on the path to the fulfillment of one's potential as a human being.

The ecstasy of the outcome

When the individual bindles, the individual's desired bodily form is delivered to the individual by the creative process. It arrives as if delivered from an outside source.

It is as simple as this: One day the individual wakes up and discovers that the desired outcome has materialized.

The ecstasy of the ripple effects of self-mastery

Through the ritual of bindling, the individual deliberately creates the powerful psychospiritual condition of self-mastery and thereby activates an automatic, inner psychospiritual process whereby the psyche and the life of the individual become transformed in their entirety.

All kinds of new possibilities begin to open up in the life of the individual, and the individual becomes empowered and insightful in finding new ways to live life to its fullest and to fulfill the potential of the self.

The ecstasy of containment

Bindling is a technique that provides the individual with a means of placing a limitation on the self. Limits in fact are essential for the experiencing of true indulgence. The placement of a limitation on the self makes it possible for the individual to experience deep, limitless, infinite ecstasy.

The psyche actually craves limits. When the individual has a means of placing a limitation on the self, the psyche feels enwombed, cared for, and contained. It is able to relax fully and becomes open and receptive to the full experiencing of pleasure. When the psyche feels contained, it functions more adaptively and responds more adaptively to all situations in life.

The ecstasy of altered consciousness

Bindling facilitates the deepest possible alteration of consciousness in that it facilitates the individual entering into and experiencing the ecstatic psychospiritual condition of paradoxical mindful mindlessness (see separate section on this for a full description of this condition).

When the individual experiences paradoxical mindful mindlessness while bindling, all of the other levels of process-reinforcing ecstasy that we have reviewed here are deepened and enhanced to levels that go far beyond the ordinary bounds of human experience.

The ecstasy of freedom

The individual who bindles achieves complete freedom from ever again having to be concerned about the task of releasing excess weight and permanently maintaining desired bodily form. This task gets turned over entirely to the creative process.

The individual then becomes free to experience the ecstasy of the creative process of life itself.

41

So it is then that in the ritual of bindling, effortlessness is achieved by means of magic and ecstasy.

The magic aspect of the effortlessness of the bindling ritual is manifested in the individual simply creating the powerful psychospiritual condition of self-mastery, and thereby turning over the task of releasing excess weight and permanently maintaining desired bodily form to the creative process as it is manifested in the deeper levels of the psyche.

The ecstasy aspect of the effortlessness of the bindling ritual is manifested in the multiple levels of ecstasy that the bindling ritual generates, which reinforce and energize the ongoing bindling process.

Effortlessness: Other ways bindling is effortless

Magic and ecstasy thus are the most basic, foundational aspects of the effortlessness of bindling. Other ways in which bindling is effortless are as follows:

Bindling is effortless in that it is a simple, once-daily, one day at a time, day-by-day process. While bindling, there is never any need to think or be concerned about what to eat next week or even the day after tomorrow. The individual who bindles remains fully present in the current day-night-day cycle.

Bindling is effortless in that it is fully amenable to the unique contours of the life of the individual. Bindling continues to be effective through all different kinds of eating phases and eating situations, and continues to exert its effects in the psyche even as the actual contents of one's diet change and evolve. Bindling is amenable to meals eaten alone, with others, while traveling, and in any other situation.

Bindling is effortless in that the individual who bindles can superimpose any other diet upon the bindling process. Whereas most diets are diets of content, bindling is a diet of process. Other diets are the paint, and bindling is the canvas. The individual who bindles possesses a technique for deliberately trying out different types of diets and creating one's own.

Bindling is effortless in that the individual who bindles is able to honor cravings in a way that is much more gratifying than willy nilly efforts to satisfy cravings. The individual who bindles possesses a specific technique for deliberately identifying deep cravings and systematically honoring them (we will discuss how to do this in greater detail in the How to Bindle chapter).

Bindling is effortless in that it allows for interpersonal invisibility. There is never any need to say to another person, "I am on a diet," unless the individual wishes to do so.

Bindling is effortless in that it is invisible timewise, and actually frees up time and energy in the life of the individual. Time that was previously spent ruminating about what to eat, pacing back and forth to the fridge, gazing into the fridge, etc.—all of that time gets reduced to a few-minutes-daily ritual. The time and energy that thus become freed up in the life of the individual are a resource that may then be channelized into whatever sorts of dreams, pursuits, passions, and so on, that the individual may have been harboring for all these years.

Bindling is effortless in that it slashes food expenses. Individuals who feel financially insecure may in fact be inclined to spend excess amounts of money on food and to acquire excess weight due to being in a continual cycle of feast or famine. The individual who bindles is able to get right down to looking at the foods that are available and designating specific foods to be received into the body. This process reassures the psyche that it is being well taken care of, prevents impulsive spending on food excess, puts extra money into the pocket of the individual, and keeps the individual on course to receive the desired outcome. Also, because the individual who bindles is in the powerful psychospiritual condition of self-mastery, the individual sees and experiences the world differently, and is therefore better equipped to formulate strategies for transforming one's station in life and thereby entering into a condition of financial confidence.

Paradox

Effective ritual is based in paradox; the individual simply positions or aligns the self in such a way that the creative process delivers to the individual the desired outcome, effortlessly, as if from an outside source.

Effortlessness
|
|
|
|
|
|
|
|
Paradox

The easiest way for us to begin to understand the paradox of effortlessness is to consider the mystery of dreaming. When we go to sleep and dream, we experience the paradox of effortlessness in its most direct, concentrated form.

Everything about dreaming is both effortless and paradoxical.

Dreaming is effortless in that the individual simply turns the self in to sleep . . . and then the dreaming occurs.

Dreaming is paradoxical in that paradox is paramount in the structure and content of dreams. Paradox is the basic organizing principle of the dreaming process, and dreams are filled with paradoxical material.

When we go to sleep and dream, we enter into the place of dreaming, which is a manifestation of the creative process within the psyche of the individual. In the place of dreaming we experience paradoxical phenomena that go completely outside the ordinary bounds of human experience.

When we enter into the place of dreaming, we experience a direct, unfiltered encounter with the divine mystery that is the creative process.

As we delve deeper and deeper into this divine mystery, we discover the deepest and most accurate truths that are available to us.

As we delve deeper and deeper into these deepest, innermost truths, we discover that paradox is the most basic, fundamental quality of these deepest, innermost truths.

Paradox is at the heart of the divine mystery that is the creative process. It is through paradox that the magic and power of the creative process are manifested in their fullness.

The ritual of bindling brings the individual into an optimal alignment with paradox, such that the individual begins to tap into the deeper magic and power of paradox—and therefore to tap into the deeper magic and power of the divine mystery that is the creative process.

Next

Next we will explore paradoxical detached attachment and paradoxical mindful mindlessness.

Paradoxical detached attachment refers to one's basic stance or approach to the bindling process, and paradoxical mindful mindlessness refers to the deep alteration of consciousness that is facilitated by the ritual of bindling.

Then we will take a break and clear the slate by considering the concept of dieting as an art form, and the way in which this concept is embodied in the ritual of bindling.

Then we will step into the process.

Paradoxical Detached Attachment

In the ritual of bindling, the individual simply positions or aligns the self in such a way that the task of effortlessly releasing excess weight and permanently maintaining one's desired bodily form gets turned over to the creative process as it is manifested in the deeper levels of the psyche. The creative process delivers this desired outcome to the individual as quickly and as effectively as is possible when the individual stays out of the way of the creative process and maintains a clear and open path through which the creative process is able to operate.

The way in which the individual stays out of the way of the creative process while bindling, so that the creative process has a clear and open path wherein it is able to deliver the desired outcome to the individual, is by dwelling entirely in ecstasy and desire, i.e., by dwelling entirely in (a) the ecstasy that is generated by the ongoing bindling process and in (b) the individual's desire for the outcome.

The easiest and most effective way to dwell entirely in ecstasy and desire on an ongoing basis while bindling is to approach the bindling ritual with a stance of paradoxical detached attachment. To approach the bindling ritual with a stance of paradoxical detached attachment involves simply entering into the sacred space of self-mastery through the Three-Day Initiation Cycle, and then simply allowing oneself to become deeply drawn into a deeply ecstatic attachment with the bindling process. This deep level of attachment and engagement between the individual and the process forms on its own while the individual focuses simply on remaining in the sacred space of self-mastery and dwelling entirely in one's desire for the outcome and in the multiple levels of ecstasy that the bindling ritual generates.

While this deep level of attachment forms between the individual and the process, the individual allows the attachment to form at the deepest possible level by deliberately detaching from anything that could possibly get in the way of the formation of the attachment. Specifically, the individual deliberately detaches from taking the bindling process too seriously, and deliberately detaches from any pushing or pulling of the self as the bindling process develops. In this way, the individual stays completely out of the way of the creative process and gives it the space it needs to materialize the desired outcome.

If at any point the individual begins to take the process too seriously or to become overly emotional about it, the individual simply redirects this energy into the basic rote repetition of the daily bindling ritual, as described in the How to Bindle chapter.

If at any point the individual begins to get into pushing or pulling of the self in the bindling process, the individual simply releases the unnecessary pressure and refocuses attention on desiring the outcome and enjoying the multiple levels of process-reinforcing ecstasy.

Enfolding All Energy Into the Task

To approach the ritual of bindling with a stance of paradoxical detached attachment is to become engaged with the ongoing bindling process, to just continue along with it, and at the same time to deliberately detach from taking it too seriously or getting overly emotional about it. Instead, the individual relaxes fully into the task, releases all tension and allows the self to become fully engaged with the task.

In paradoxical detached attachment, the individual gently holds the image of the desired outcome in mind and remains gently engaged with the task. At the same time, the individual refuses to become frantic, desperate, or eager about getting to the end point. Instead, the individual channelizes all energy into becoming fully engaged with the direct sensorial experience of moving along through all the steps and stages of the process. Any kind of emotionality that arises gets redirected into the task itself, into the individual's engagement with the task and the process of continuing along with it. Then, while in this task-connected space, the individual simply witnesses as the desired outcome materializes.

Paradoxical detached attachment is the way to fall in love with the journey itself, and not just the destination or the outcome. When we bindle we do value the outcome highly, and the outcome does in fact become materialized. However, this happens as a function of the individual slowing things down and relaxing fully into the creative process of having the desired outcome delivered to the self.

When we focus all of our attention into a valued creative process, everything else corrects itself by default. Continually bringing our attention back to the creative process in which we are presently engaged turns over all of our unresolved challenges to the creative process as it is manifested in the deeper levels of the psyche. Then, within the deeper levels of the psyche, the creative process comes up with the best possible ways for all of our challenges to be overcome.

Relaxing oneself into the process is a gentle, gradual, ongoing process. Over time the internal temper tantrums and dramatics get swallowed up and absorbed into the grand ocean of the infinite. We become soothed as we become pulled into the creative process, as we allow our attention to gently flow into the ecstatic process of gently holding the desired outcome in mind while remaining gently engaged with the task that leads to the desired outcome.

Detaching From Pushing or Pulling

To approach bindling with a stance of paradoxical detached attachment is to allow one's full motivation for participation in bindling to arise from one's innate desire to experience the desired outcome and the various levels of process-reinforcing ecstasy—and to deliberately detach from any other possible motivation for engaging in the process.

The individual who bindles develops extraordinary discipline in a paradoxically effortless manner, and the power of this discipline ripples out into and transforms all aspects of the life of the individual. The discipline that emerges from the process of bindling is deeper and more powerful than any other possible form of discipline because of the fact that it arises from the innate manifestation of the divine within the individual, i.e., from the individual's innate desiring process. There is no form of discipline that is more powerful than discipline that is innately desired, for in innately desired discipline the full power of the creative process becomes embodied and manifested.

The individual uses the bindling ritual to create the powerful psychospiritual condition of self-mastery because the individual innately desires to do so, because the process itself feels good and because the desired outcome is truly desired. To develop the discipline of self-mastery based not on desire but instead based on the idea that one "should" develop such discipline is a way of blocking the innate flowing process of desire, and brings the individual into an effortful trudging along in a dreary sense of obligation. The individual who trudges along in this way loses sight of the many options and possibilities that are continually spread out before us, enters into a condition of stuckness and inertia, and becomes unwilling to accept self and others as is.

To approach bindling with the highly adaptive stance of paradoxical detached attachment is to deliberately detach from any sense that bindling is something that is required of the self or that it is something that the individual "should" do. So then if at any point the individual begins to think of bindling as an obligation (e.g., "I have to," "I should," "I need to," etc.), the individual deliberately detaches from this sort of thinking by just letting go of it and relaxing into the basic stance of allowing all motivation for bindling to arise entirely from the divine, i.e., to arise from the innate, ongoing flowing process of desire as it emerges from within the self. In this way, the individual stays completely out of the way of the creative process, and the creative process then has a clear and open path through which it is able to deliver the desired outcome to the individual as quickly and as effectively as is possible.

Paradoxical Mindful Mindlessness

The ritual of bindling is rewarding to the individual in that it activates a deep, underlying process wherein the individual's desired bodily form materializes, and also because—as a function of the activation of this deep, underlying process—the psyche and life of the individual become transformed in their entirety.

In addition to all of these highly rewarding outcomes of the bindling process, bindling is rewarding to the individual in that it invokes the most profound alteration of consciousness wherein the individual experiences the psychospiritual condition of paradoxical mindful mindlessness.

Paradoxical mindful mindlessness is mystic experience, in which the individual experiences direct contact, direct communion, and direct relationship with the divine mystery that is the creative process.

Paradoxical mindful mindlessness is the ultimate psychospiritual condition because it is a condition of magic and ecstasy. The individual who enters into this condition experiences the magic of receiving fully formed solutions to all of life's challenges, and experiences the deepest and most profound levels of ecstasy that are possible to be experienced.

All ritual, including bindling, is a potential means of experiencing the condition of paradoxical mindful mindlessness. Ritual that is most effective in bringing the individual into this psychospiritual condition is (a) simple, (b) rote or repetitious, and (c) absorbs the full attention and energy of the individual.

The individual enters into the condition of paradoxical mindful mindlessness by filling the mind entirely with the ritual and all of its nuances in their fullness. This complete filling of the mind facilitates a paradoxical emptying and clearing out of the mind.

In paradoxical mindful mindlessness, the mind becomes as it were a blank canvas, and everything else just kind of falls off and disappears. The individual becomes fully absorbed in the delights of the ritual and experiences sort of a soothing self-hypnosis, an emptying out of the psyche that facilitates the deepest possible levels of ecstasy and bliss.

Paradoxical mindful mindlessness deepens the individual's sensorial experience of all of the multiple levels of ecstasy that are generated by the bindling process. It brings the individual into a condition of deeper receptivity and sensitivity to all of life's pleasures. Paradoxical mindful mindlessness is better than any drug, with deeper and longer lasting effects, and no crash.

Paradoxical mindful mindlessness is the state of mind of a child, a condition of complete freedom in which the individual directly experiences the possibilities of the infinite. In this state of consciousness there is no real sense of past, present, and future; rather, there is only an eternally present, magic now.

Paradoxical mindful mindlessness brings the mind to the place of dreaming, which is a manifestation of the creative process in the psyche of the individual. The place of dreaming is the same place the mind goes to when it experiences dreams in sleep. When the individual deliberately invokes the condition of paradoxical mindful mindlessness, it is as if the individual is dreaming while awake. This is the means whereby the individual is able to deliberately interact with the divine and to participate in magic in waking life. When the individual goes to the place of dreaming while awake, the challenges of life work themselves out on their own. The individual may playfully mull over challenges while in the condition of paradoxical mindful mindlessness, as this is part of the challenge-solving process that occurs once the individual has effectively cleared the slate: Potential solutions to a challenge begin to dance around on the blank canvas of the mind, and because the individual is focused mainly on the present-moment ritual—rather than on the challenges directly—the individual is able to maintain a stance of paradoxical detached attachment to the challenges. So the individual may playfully consider possible solutions to the challenges, but ultimately keeps the focus on the ritual at hand, on clearing the slate, and on ecstasy. Then, just when the individual least expects it—perhaps on a different day, while doing who knows what—there appears in the mind a complete, fully formed solution to the challenge. It appears there on its own, seemingly by magic. In fact, it is an experience of true magic.

Any type of simple, repetitive, absorbing ritual is effective in bringing the individual into the condition of paradoxical mindful mindlessness and thus into direct contact with the place of dreaming. This could be any type of creative project, or even mundane tasks like doing the dishes or taking a shower. Cooking is highly conducive to the condition of paradoxical mindful mindlessness, and is an excellent way for the individual who bindles to become more directly acquainted with the nuances of various foods.

The individual who develops an appreciation for the psychospiritual condition of paradoxical mindful mindlessness becomes empowered to discover the hidden ecstasy potential of even the most seemingly unlikely of mundane tasks, such as paying the bills or doing the laundry. This doesn't mean that it is always easy to get started on such activities, but the fact remains that such activities do have the potential to bring the mind of the individual to another place, to the place of dreaming.

Listening to a musical recording while participating in a simple, rote, absorbing task can be a particularly magical experience that brings the individual along on a journey through the place of dreaming. And then sometimes too it can be very rewarding to participate in an extremely simple, rote, absorbing activity in absolute silence, accompanied only by the music of the subtler sounds that surround us.

Paradoxical mindful mindlessness is paradoxical because the emptying of the mind is achieved by filling the mind entirely, by allowing it to become fully absorbed in the task of the present moment. This is why it is almost never a good idea to just kind of sit around and think in an aimless sort of way, in a state of entropy. It is almost always better for the psyche to have some type of deliberate activity or ritual into which attention can be gently directed. This can be something as simple as a breathing meditation, in which the individual allows the entirety of mental attention to become fully absorbed in the process of observing the in breath, the out breath, the in breath, and the out breath . . . and on and on it goes, of the ongoing breathing process.

Emptying the mind is essential both for the experiencing of ecstasy and for facilitating the creative process as it delivers the desired outcome to the individual. When the individual who bindles deliberately keeps the bindling ritual as effortless as is possible, this facilitates the ongoing mind-emptying process, keeps the individual out of the way of the creative process, and facilitates the creative process in delivering the desired outcome to the individual as quickly and as effectively as is possible.

In fact, becoming comfortable with emptiness is a key psychospiritual process that facilitates effortless releasing of excess weight and permanent maintenance of desired bodily form. The body holds onto excess weight when it has spent years believing that fulfillment is good and that emptiness is bad. The healing process begins once the individual begins to fall in love with emptiness, with the void, with moments of silence and solitude and quiet meditation. As the individual gradually begins to discover the deeper levels of ecstasy hidden inside emptiness, the body itself begins to relax and let go of the excess weight it had been retaining.

The condition of paradoxical mindful mindlessness reaches peak levels of ecstasy, levels of ecstasy that go completely outside the ordinary bounds of human experience, when the individual experiences this condition (a) in the context of the condition of self-mastery and (b) while the individual is engaged with a goal. The individual who bindles experiences both of these factors in that the individual who bindles deliberately creates the condition of self-mastery by bindling, and at the same time becomes engaged with the goal of effortlessly releasing excess weight and permanently maintaining desired bodily form. Therefore, bindling has the potential to bring into the life of the individual levels of ecstasy that go completely outside the ordinary bounds of human experience.

Bindling has the basic characteristics of a ritual that is effective in facilitating the condition of paradoxical mindful mindlessness: It is simple, repetitive (repeated daily), and absorbs the full attention of the individual for a few minutes each day. Also, the qualities of mindfulness and mindlessness are embedded in the bindling ritual itself: The individual spends a few minutes of mindful focus on the daily bindling ritual, and then releases it. During the rest of the day the individual simply gets on with the activities of daily life.

Bindling also facilitates paradoxical mindful mindlessness in that it keeps the individual grounded in the present moment: Bindling keeps the individual focused simply on the current day-night-day cycle of planet Earth as it rotates around its Sun. The individual may put some special eating occasions on the calendar for upcoming days, weeks, or months, but the actual eating plans for these occasions are not deliberately specified until the day prior. In this way, the individual remains deeply grounded in and connected with the creative process as it is occurring in the present moment, in the current day-night-day cycle, and is able to keep the mind emptied of unnecessary concern about the past and the future.

74

Because the individual who bindles becomes freed from having to think about what to eat except during the brief, few-minutes-daily bindling ritual, time and energy become freed up in the psyche, and the individual experiences a newfound opportunity to begin to explore the possibilities of life and of human potential. The individual may therefore begin to think about new projects, new hobbies, new goals, new adventures, and so on.

Because the individual who bindles is facilitating in the psyche a gradually increasing condition of paradoxical mindful mindlessness, the process of exploring new ideas and possibilities occurs in a whole new way. The individual is able to reflect on and engage with possibilities and ideas with a sense of playful detachment, with a stance of paradoxical detached attachment wherein the individual engages with the ideas without ever taking them too seriously. This paradoxical stance actually allows the ideas to be crafted and re-crafted by the deeper magic of the creative process, and keeps the individual out of the way as this occurs.

The real beauty though of bindling is that while the individual who bindles is able to playfully explore new possibilities and ideas on the blank mental canvas of paradoxical mindful mindlessness, this playful exploratory process occurs (a) in the context of the powerful psychospiritual condition of self-mastery and (b) in the presence of a valued goal (i.e., effortless releasing of excess weight and permanent maintenance of desired bodily form). In this unique context, the solution providing that is facilitated by paradoxical mindful mindlessness gets thrown into a whole new league, and into a whole new ball game altogether. This solution providing that is facilitated by paradoxical mindful mindlessness, which is normally focused on how to get the individual out of a jam, becomes redirected into figuring out how to fulfill the life potential of the individual.

This is why experiencing paradoxical mindful mindlessness in the context of self-mastery and in the presence of a goal is the utmost in magic and ecstasy: The place of dreaming becomes fully facilitated in exerting its full effects in the life of the individual, and the individual experiences a deeper level of engagement with the creative process and its ever-deepening levels of ecstasy.

In summary, the individual who bindles begins the bindling process with the goal of effortlessly releasing excess weight and permanently maintaining desired bodily form. The bindling process facilitates the individual entering into the psychospiritual condition of paradoxical mindful mindlessness, which facilitates the individual in playfully considering new ideas and new goals to pursue. Because the individual is playfully considering these ideas while in the powerful psychospiritual condition of self-mastery and in the presence of a goal (i.e., the original goal of releasing excess weight and permanently maintaining desired bodily form), the place of dreaming becomes facilitated in formulating and presenting to the individual simple next steps to take in pursuing one or more new goals. One important aspect of this process is that the place of dreaming becomes facilitated in helping the individual to figure out the specific goals that will be most effective in tickling the innermost fancy of the psyche.

Simply having a valued goal—no matter what the goal may be—is the single most important factor in the well-being of the psyche. The reason for this is that humans are manifestations of the creative process, and as such, will only ever be content while creating in one way or another. Therefore, becoming engaged with

76

a desired goal is simply a way of becoming atoned with one's innately divine nature as a manifestation of the creative process. The embracing of a goal that is innately desired by the individual is not at all an "adding on" of an assignment to the self. The embracing of a goal that is innately desired is, in fact, a task of releasing and emptying, i.e., releasing and emptying out whatever it may be that is keeping the individual stuck and blocked from manifesting the innate flowing of the creative process as it continually seeks to express itself in the life of the individual.

The path between where the individual is now and a desired goal—whatever the goal may be—need not be clear. Simply having a goal facilitates the well-being of the psyche and unblocks its true nature as a manifestation of the creative process. In fact, half the fun is observing and witnessing as the creative process itself figures out, on the individual's behalf, how the individual is going to receive the goal. In the case of bindling, the task of the individual is simply to embrace the ritual, to turn over the task of delivering the desired outcome to the creative process as it is manifested in the deeper levels of the psyche, and to dwell entirely in one's desire for the outcome and in the multiple levels of process-reinforcing ecstasy.

Dieting as an Art Form

Our hunter-gatherer ancestors used ritual for the purpose of receiving food from the creative process. With the eventual advent of agriculture, our more recent ancestors continued to use ritual for the purpose of receiving food from the creative process, but did so in a manner that was characterized by additional forethought, planning, calculation, and deliberation. This advanced approach to ritualization was remarkably effective and to this day is continuing to be refined and advanced to ever-increasing levels of productivity.

In fact, agriculture has become so successful that we now live in a world in which some individuals have access to far more food than is necessary to survive. For individuals who have such access to food excess, there is a need for ritual to evolve further still, to provide a way for such individuals to set limitations on their intake of the food that is available to them, while still being able to fully enjoy the pleasures of eating.

Bindling serves this purpose in the life of the individual. It allows the individual to fully experiment with and explore the multiplicity of food options that are available in our increasingly globalized, interconnected world, and to simultaneously experience one's desired bodily form.

Bindling accomplishes this by building on the forethought, planning, calculation, and deliberation of agriculture, but applies these qualities to the process of limiting one's intake of the abundance that agriculture has produced.

The individual who bindles approaches dieting not as an obligation, but rather as an art form, as a creative process, as a technique of ecstasy.

When the individual approaches dieting as an art form, it is the individual's own body that is the creative medium. Thinking of dieting in this way assists the individual in recognizing that the body itself is a manifestation of the creative process, and as such it is divine and sacred. Once the individual is able to recognize that the body is a manifestation of the divine, then the natural consequence of this recognition is that the individual desires only to take good care of the body, to tend to it and honor it and to respect its innate holiness.

We tend to think of art as something that exists outside the self, outside the body, because we tend to think of the divine as something that exists outside the self and outside the body. Approaching dieting as an art form entails recognizing that spirit and flesh are one and the same, and that the body is a manifestation of the divine, a manifestation of the creative process. To see ourselves as we truly are, for the self to become fully transparent to the self, our first task is to see through and transcend the illusion of separateness.

Seeing through the illusion of separateness and approaching dieting as an art form facilitates the individual in maintaining a stance of neutrality in regard to the body as a creative medium. The individual who participates in the bindling ritual is able to view the body as a manifestation of the divine that is, simultaneously, a mere accretion of elements, a bodily form that is continuous with all of the elements in the universe in all of their manifested forms and conditions.

The concept of dieting as an art form provides the individual with a creative path that is balanced between the extremes of the starving artist of Romanticism and the over-indulgent, self-destructive artist of the 20th century. The individual who bindles is an indulging artist, one who appreciates and values pleasure and yet who understands that pleasure and ecstasy are really only possible when the individual has a means of containing the self and experiencing reasonable limits.

Approaching dieting as an art form is, above all else, the most effective way to approach dieting. It keeps the focus on the process of diet rather than on its contents, because the process is more important than the contents. When the individual bindles, the individual becomes engaged with a process in which the actual contents of one's diet evolve adaptively, on their own, as a function of the creative process. Bindling simply creates the crucible in which this happens.

So the art of bindling then is to focus simply on creating the crucible, i.e., creating the powerful psychospiritual condition of self-mastery in as effortless a manner as is possible, and to turn over all the rest to the creative process as it is manifested in the deeper levels of the psyche. And to then take in a deep breath . . . and let out a huge sigh of relief . . . and to dwell entirely in ecstasy and desire.

THE *PROCESS*

The remainder of this book consists of a series of process chapters. The first of these process chapters, How to Bindle, provides specific, detailed instructions on how to participate in the ritual of bindling.

In the subsequent process chapters, we explore the deeper, underlying psychospiritual process that is activated by the ritual of bindling — the deeper, internal process that leads to the materialization of the individual's desired bodily form.

Then, at the end of the book, we will proceed with the Three-Day Initiation Cycle. Through the Three-Day Initiation Cycle, we will initiate our participation in the bindling ritual and will thereby enter into the sacred space of self-mastery.

Forms that are used for the Three-Day Initiation Cycle and 100 days of bindling are provided at the end of the Three-Day Initiation Cycle chapter.

How to Bindle   →   Self-
Mastery   →

Transformation
of Self → Condition of
Inevitability → Desired
Outcome

The process chapters are as follows:

How to Bindle

We will begin in the How to Bindle chapter with an overview of the basic logistics of the ritual of bindling.

In this chapter we will also discuss some of the ways in which the bindling ritual is likely to evolve over time.

Also in this chapter we will explore some of the ways in which bindling can enhance and deepen one's ongoing experience of the ecstasy of eating.

Note that the purpose of the How to Bindle chapter is simply for soaking in the basics of the bindling process. We will actually get started with bindling at the end of the book, in the Three-Day Initiation Cycle chapter.

Self-Mastery

In the Self-Mastery chapter, we will explore the powerful psychospiritual condition of self-mastery that is created by the bindling ritual, and the pivotal role of this condition in the dieting process.

In this chapter we will also explore the deeper psychospiritual process of claiming ownership of self and its relation to the condition of self-mastery.

Transformation of Self

In the Transformation of Self chapter, we will explore the intricacies of the deeper, underlying, automatic transformation of self process that is activated once the individual enters into the sacred space of self-mastery, i.e., the process wherein the psyche and the life of the individual come to be transformed in their entirety.

As we explore the intricacies of the transformation of self process, we will also explore the intricacies of ecstasy and desire, because it is in dwelling entirely in ecstasy and desire that the individual is able to stay completely out of the way of the creative process as it carries out the transformation of self.

Condition of Inevitability

In the Condition of Inevitability chapter, we will explore how to gently accelerate the momentum of the underlying transformation of self process such that the individual enters into the condition of inevitability—the condition in which the desired outcome becomes inevitable and materializes—as quickly and as effectively as is possible.

Specifically, in this chapter we will discuss how to channelize one's innate desiring process through the technique of paradoxical dual flooding so as to enter into the condition of inevitability as quickly and as effectively as is possible.

This chapter includes a discussion of how to use power objects to facilitate the paradoxical dual flooding process. Also, it includes a discussion of how to allow one's personal spaces to become transformed such that the paradoxical dual flooding process fully engulfs the psyche.

Desired Outcome

In the Desired Outcome chapter, we will explore the experience of the desired outcome becoming fully materialized and manifested in the life of the individual.

In this chapter, we will discuss how to fully receive and integrate the desired outcome into one's life.

In the Desired Outcome chapter we will also explore ways in which the ritual of bindling facilitates an effortless rippling out of increased movement and exercising of the body.

Also, in this chapter we will go into a deeper exploration of the creative process itself. Specifically, we will explore some of the ways in which the ritual of bindling facilitates the individual in developing a personal creative path wherein the individual is able to experience the deepest possible ongoing communion with the creative process.

Three-Day Initiation Cycle

In the Three-Day Initiation Cycle chapter, we will review the basics of how to bindle (i.e., the basic information from the How to Bindle chapter) and will ritually enter into the sacred space of self-mastery.

How to Bindle

In the ritual of bindling, the individual focuses simply on deliberately creating the powerful psychospiritual condition of self-mastery, and thereby turns over the task of releasing excess weight and permanently maintaining one's desired bodily form to the creative process as it is manifested in the deeper levels of the psyche.

The individual creates the powerful psychospiritual condition of self-mastery by creating a repeated daily pattern of (a) obtaining and documenting food to be eaten one day in advance and (b) following through with this plan on the designated day.

The key to an effective, ecstatic bindling process is to continually keep it as simple and as effortless as possible, and really, just to have fun with the process, to approach it with a spirit of play.

The daily bindling ritual involves the completion of a one-page form. A set of bindling forms is provided in this book, at the end of the Three-Day Initiation Cycle chapter.

Unboxing Press also publishes booklets of bindling forms that are available for purchase separately. These separately published booklets are available in two formats, the basic version and the advanced version.

> *Basic Forms.* The basic version is identical to the set of bindling forms included in this book (at the end of the Three-Day Initiation Cycle chapter). These basic forms include forms for the Three-Day Initiation Cycle and 100 days of bindling. Booklets of basic forms can be identified by one black horizontal stripe that wraps around the upper portion of the booklet cover.

> *Advanced Forms.* The advanced version is for individuals who have been initiated into the sacred space of self-mastery and have remained within that space for 100 days. The advanced forms are mostly identical to the basic forms; the one difference is that the advanced forms do not include forms for the initiation process. Initiated individuals may use the advanced forms for Days 101 to 200, Days 201 to 300, and so on. Booklets of advanced forms can be identified by two black horizontal stripes that wrap around the upper portion of the booklet cover.

The daily bindling ritual is a daily repetition of a simple series of tasks that are set into motion during the Three-Day Initiation Cycle. The easiest way to understand how the bindling ritual works is to first understand how the Three-Day Initiation Cycle works.

Therefore, in this chapter, we will review the basic logistics of the Three-Day Initiation Cycle. Keep in mind though that the purpose of this chapter is simply for soaking in the basics of how to bindle. We will review these basics again when we ritually enter into the sacred space of self-mastery in the Three-Day Initiation Cycle chapter.

The three days in the Three-Day Initiation Cycle are (1) the Pre-Liminal Day, (2) the Liminal Day, and (3) the Initiation Day. Note that in the ritual of bindling, days are divided by sleep cycles (not from midnight to midnight).

Each of these three days is represented by a separate one-page form (see the first three pages of the forms that are located at the end of the Three-Day Initiation Cycle chapter). The forms for each of the three days in the Three-Day Initiation Cycle are identified as follows:

> *Pre-Liminal Day.* The form for the Pre-Liminal Day is indicated by the words "*PRE-LIMINAL* DAY" that appear at the top of the form.

Liminal Day. The form for the Liminal Day is indicated by the words *"LIMINAL* DAY" that appear at the top of the form.

Initiation Day. The form for the Initiation Day appears on the page immediately following the page on which the form for the Liminal Day appears. The form for the Initiation Day is indicated by the image of a laurel wreath that appears at the top of the form.

The Initiation Day form symbolizes entry into the sacred space of self-mastery. All subsequent forms are identical to the Initiation Day form, and thus symbolize ongoing continuation of the sacred space of self-mastery.

The tasks completed on each of the three days in the Three-Day Initiation Cycle are as follows:

PRE-LIMINAL DAY

1. Write today's date in YYMMDD format in the lower right-hand corner of the Pre-Liminal Day form.

2. Write tomorrow's date in the lower right-hand corner of the Liminal Day form.

3. Select a series of food items to be eaten on the Liminal Day. These items will be listed on the Liminal Day form.

    In the food selection process, make sure that it will be ridiculously easy to follow through with the designated plan. This is not the time to place any sort of unnecessary challenge on the self. Just following through with a designated plan is challenge enough, in and of itself.

    In coming up with a plan, it may be helpful to sketch out ideas on a separate piece of paper or in an electronic document.

    Select food items based on the following three categories:

Unlimited

The unlimited category is for food items that the individual wishes to be able to consume in unlimited amounts. These are items that the individual is confident will not impede the process of effortlessly releasing excess weight and permanently maintaining desired bodily form, regardless of amounts consumed.

The individual may wish to think of some unlimited items as treats. Unlimited items do not need to be obtained prior to the Liminal Day, as the individual is free to consume unlimited items in any amount (including "none") on the Liminal Day.

Obtained

The obtained category is the main category in the bindling ritual, and allows for the highest level of specificity. Items that are listed in the obtained category on the Liminal Day form are obtained on the Pre-Liminal Day; in other words, they are obtained one day in advance. It is in the obtained category that the creative process is able to do the majority of its work.

Ritualized

The ritualized category is for various types of special eating occasions, such as social eating rituals, in which the individual does not necessarily specify the precise foods that will be eaten, but rather specifies participation in a specific eating ritual. The ritualized category allows for more spontaneous eating experiences that are tethered to a specific eating ritual (e.g., a wedding, a meal at a restaurant, etc.). Any number of ritualized eating occasions (including "none") can be specified for any specific day.

Obtained alternate plan

For any eating ritual that is specified in the ritualized category, the individual also includes an obtained alternate plan. The obtained alternate plan is the backup plan of the specific foods to be eaten in case the planned eating ritual falls through, for whatever reason.

Items in the obtained alternate plan are similar to items listed in the main "obtained" category: They are listed in specific amounts, and are obtained one day in advance.

It is not necessary to include items in all three categories (i.e., unlimited, obtained, and ritualized) on the plan for any given day. The key to success is to focus the majority of one's attention on the obtained category, as it is in this category that the creative process is able to carry out the majority of its work.

The most important thing to keep in mind is that in the ritual of bindling, the main task of the individual is simply to create and maintain the sacred space of self-mastery. While it is true that self-mastery is a powerful psychospiritual condition, the key to accessing its full potential is to always make it ridiculously easy to follow through with the designated plan.

This is the paradox of effortlessness. When the individual keeps the bindling process effortless, the psyche becomes increasingly disciplined on its own, without any pushing or pulling of the self.

4. After the items to be eaten on the Liminal Day have been selected, write out the selected plan on the Liminal Day form.

   Keep this as effortless as possible by using easily understood abbreviations and shorthand. Specific instructions for each of the three categories are as follows:

   Unlimited

   Write out the names of any foods to be permitted in unlimited amounts on the Liminal Day.

   Obtained

   Write out the (a) names and (b) specific amounts of foods designated to be eaten on the Liminal Day.

Ritualized

For any ritualized eating occasion, write out both (a) a description of the bounds of the eating occasion and (b) the obtained alternate plan, as follows:

Bounds of the eating occasion

Write out a specific description of the bounds of the eating occasion. The most simple way to do this is to write, "Whatever I wish to eat at . . .," and then specify the occasion.

Additional limitations and/or specifications may be included in the description, but it is important to not set oneself up for a situation in which one's intended plan might be compromised. For example, if an individual were to specify that exactly one plate of food is to be eaten at a particular social eating event, others who are present at the event may unknowingly compromise this person's plan by sampling from the person's plate, possibly even without asking for permission to do so.

The key to success is to chart out a path for oneself in which the follow-through is effortless and inevitable. Therefore, it is best to define the bounds of a ritualized eating occasion in such a way that the individual will be able to fully relax and enjoy the occasion, and rest assured that the plan is being carried out effortlessly and as intended.

Obtained alternate plan

After the description of the bounds of the eating occasion, write "Alt.:" followed by the (a) names and (b) specific amounts of foods designated to be eaten in case the eating occasion falls through, for whatever reason.

5. After the selected plan for the Liminal Day has been finalized and written out on the Liminal Day form, check off the OBT and DOC boxes on the Pre-Liminal Day form.

OBT box

Checking off the OBT box on the Pre-Liminal Day form indicates that all of the items listed as obtained on the Liminal Day form have been obtained.

This refers to both (a) items in the main obtained category and (b) items obtained as alternate (i.e., backup) for anything planned in the ritualized category.

DOC box

Checking off the DOC box on the Pre-Liminal Day form indicates that the full eating plan for the Liminal Day has been documented (i.e., written out) on the Liminal Day form.

Optional

A series of Ws appears in the lower left-hand corner of the Pre-Liminal Day form and all subsequent forms. These Ws are provided for individuals who wish to track their water intake in whatever way is helpful to them.

LIMINAL DAY

1. Follow through with the eating plan specified on the Liminal Day form.

2. Write tomorrow's date in the lower right-hand corner of the Initiation Day form (i.e., the form on the page following the page on which the Liminal Day form appears).

3. Select a series of food items to be eaten on the Initiation Day, in the same way that the series of food items to be eaten on the Liminal Day was selected on the Pre-Liminal Day.

   Consider including some type of celebratory item to be enjoyed on the Initiation Day.

4. Write out the selected plan on the Initiation Day form, in the same way that the selected plan for the Liminal Day was written out on the Liminal Day form, on the Pre-Liminal Day.

Make sure that all items listed as obtained have been obtained; this includes both (a) items in the main obtained category and (b) items obtained as alternate (i.e., backup) for anything planned in the ritualized category.

5. Check off the OBT and DOC boxes on the Liminal Day form.

INITIATION DAY, or Day 1

On the Initiation Day, the first task of the individual is to write the number "1" in the center of the laurel wreath at the top of the Initiation Day form. This signifies that the individual has entered into the sacred space of self-mastery. The remaining tasks on the Initiation Day are essentially the same as the tasks completed on the Liminal Day:

1. Follow through with the eating plan specified on the Initiation Day (Day 1) form.

2. Write tomorrow's date in the lower right-hand corner of the Day 2 form (i.e., the form on the page following the page on which the Initiation Day form appears).

3. Select a series of food items to be eaten on Day 2, in the same way that food items were selected one day ahead on the previous two days.

4. Write out the selected plan on the Day 2 form, in the same way that the selected plans were written out one day ahead on the previous two days.

114

Make sure that all items listed as obtained have been obtained, including both (a) items in the main obtained category and (b) items obtained as alternate (i.e., backup) for anything planned in the ritualized category.

5. Check off the OBT and DOC boxes on the Initiation Day form.

Day 2, Day 3, and on we go

The tasks completed on each subsequent day are as follows:

First, write the next consecutive day number ("2" on Day 2, "3" on Day 3, etc.) in the center of the laurel wreath at the top of the current day form (i.e., the form on which today's menu appears). This signifies continuation of the sacred space of self-mastery. Then,

1. Follow through with the eating plan as specified on the current day form.

2. Write tomorrow's date in the lower right-hand corner of the next day form (i.e., the form on the page following the page on which the current day form appears).

3. Select a series of food items to be eaten tomorrow, in the same way that food items were selected one day ahead on each day of the Three-Day Initiation Cycle.

4. Write out the selected plan on the next day form, in the same way that the selected plans were written out one day ahead on each day of the Three-Day Initiation Cycle.

   Make sure that all items listed as obtained have been obtained, including both (a) items in the main obtained category and (b) items obtained as alternate (i.e., backup) for anything planned in the ritualized category.

5. Check off the OBT and DOC boxes on the current day form.

The Daily Approach

Of the five daily bindling tasks listed above, task 1—i.e., following through with today's menu—is something that can be spread across the entire day. On the current day form, the individual may wish to check off each specific food item as it is eaten throughout the course of the day.

To keep the daily process as effortless as possible, the individual may wish to complete tasks 2, 3, 4, and 5 as early as possible each day.

117

The few daily minutes that are devoted to completing tasks 2, 3, 4, and 5 provide for the individual a sacred space in which the individual is able to experience direct communion with the creative process.

At times the individual may get really into the process of bindling and get carried away in the enjoyment of selecting and specifying foods. If this happens, great, but it is not necessary, as bindling really only requires a few minutes of focused attention, once per day.

Regardless of how much time the individual ends up spending on the daily bindling ritual, this amount of time will always be less than the amounts of time the individual used to spend (i.e., before bindling) in willy nilly food rumination.

After tasks 2, 3, 4, and 5 are completed, the individual is able to let go completely and enter into the other creative processes of the day, i.e., whatever activities the individual has planned for the day.

Other Considerations

Bindling is a technique that is flexible and amenable to whatever the personal life situation of the individual may be. Part of the pleasure of the ongoing bindling process is figuring out how to keep it going as effortlessly as is possible.

This may at times present a mild challenge to the individual, a challenge that is akin to the solving of an easy level crossword puzzle.

For example, the individual may need to figure out a convenient food storage system in which there is a clear designation and separation between (a) items that were bindled yesterday to be eaten today and (b) items that are bindled today to be eaten tomorrow.

Also, the individual who bindles will need to do whatever may be necessary—depending on one's personal living situation—to ensure that bindled food items will not be eaten by individuals who live with the individual and/or by individuals who visit.

In addition, the individual who travels often will need to figure out selections of foods that are both enjoyable and portable, that will not spoil easily, and that will pass through security checkpoints (e.g., at airports).

The Process Refines Itself

The individual who bindles focuses simply on completing the daily bindling ritual, which creates the powerful psychospiritual condition of self-mastery, and thereby turns over the task of releasing excess weight and permanently maintaining desired bodily form to the creative process as it is manifested in the deeper levels of the psyche.

119

Then, what happens over time is that the individual begins to make gradual, innately desired refinements in the bindling process. Because these refinements are innately desired, they are effortless and occur on their own, without any pushing or pulling of the self, as the process itself takes over and refines itself. The individual merely witnesses these refinements as they occur.

This automatic refinement in the bindling process is facilitated simply by the individual entering into the powerful psychospiritual condition of self-mastery, and allowing this condition to become stronger and more powerful on its own, while the individual simply continues along with the day-by-day bindling process.

As the condition of self-mastery becomes stronger and more powerful, it begins to serve as a powerful source of psychospiritual leverage within the psyche of the individual, wherein the individual becomes capable of exhibiting a most extraordinary level of discipline in a manner that is, paradoxically, completely effortless.

Something to Look Forward To

The condition of self-mastery is the main source of psychospiritual leverage experienced by the individual who bindles. Another source of leverage that the individual who bindles is able to harness is that of providing for oneself something to look forward to—specifically, by plotting out one's upcoming indulgence in treats.

The process of plotting out one's upcoming indulgence in treats, i.e., the process of making sure one always has something to look forward to, makes it so much easier to set reasonable limits on the self.

Having something to look forward to is of utmost importance in the well-being of the psyche. Treats serve as psychological oases for the individual, and like goals, treats provide the psyche with a sense of direction and thereby serve to keep the psyche going and functioning properly. Treats thus are both a necessity and a luxury, i.e., they are a necessary luxury.

Knowing that one has a treat to look forward to imbues all of life's more mundane moments with a mild thrill. Treats are special because, by definition, they are occasional. The individual deliberately inserts intervals between treats so that the treats will actually be experienced in the psyche as treats. Spacing treats out is a way of making them more special and satisfying.

For the individual who bindles, the actual definition of what a treat is is something that evolves, ebbs, and flows over time. Over time the individual may discover that one particular food item once thought of as "healthy" actually has an extraordinary ability to arouse the senses and to provide pleasure to the individual. Bindling facilitates the individual's participation in an ongoing process wherein the individual is able to deliberately explore what a treat is to the individual, and to observe the ways in which this definition evolves, ebbs, and flows within the self over time.

One of the most important services that bindling provides to the individual is that of clearing the sensory slate. As the sensory slate is cleared, the individual is able to begin to discover the hidden ecstatic potential of all kinds of seemingly mundane foods. As the individual begins to discover some of the more subtle pleasurable nuances of various "healthier" items, the individual may notice within the self a tendency to go back to certain food items again and again, to experience these food items repeatedly by placing them on the menu day after day. While these beloved, repeated foods may not necessarily be thought of as treats per se, they are similar to treats in that they provide pleasure and satisfaction to the individual.

Core menu

Once the individual begins to notice a pattern of going back to particular beloved "healthier" food items again and again, this indicates that a core menu is beginning to form in the individual's bindling process. A core menu consists of the basic food items the individual eats most of the time, and is based on the individual discovering just the right balance between (a) what the individual considers to be the healthiest foods available and (b) what the individual actually wants to eat.

The core menu may consist of just a few items or many items, and it may evolve rapidly or very slowly. It is a highly individualized process. As the core menu begins to form, the individual's bindling process becomes increasingly effortless: The individual is able to repeat favored items day after day, and to make subtle tweaks and adjustments here and there as desired.

Once the individual notices that a core menu is beginning to form in one's bindling process, the individual may then wish to become more deliberately focused on refining the core menu, as a deliberate creative process. One way of engaging with the process of refining one's core menu is to begin to study the science of diet and nutrition.

There is a lot of information about diet and nutrition that is available to be studied, and some of this information has changed and evolved—and will continue to change and evolve—over time. Bindling provides the individual with a means of grounding oneself in the midst of this plethora of evolving information. By bindling, the individual is able to make a deliberate, daily executive decision about what to put on the next day's menu, based on the individual's current understanding of diet and nutrition.

The key to success in studying the science of diet and nutrition is to approach it as an evolving, ongoing learning process in which one participates when one innately desires to do so. Most of us already have a pretty basic idea of the nutritional qualities of various foods, so there really is no need to do a bunch of additional research prior to getting started with the bindling process. Between now and whenever we finish our research— which by definition is something that is never finished—we still have to eat. So the key to success in bindling then is simply to begin now based on whatever foods we have already been habitually eating, and to then learn and refine as the process evolves.

The magic of bindling is that the simple act of making a daily executive decision about what to eat on the following day begins to naturally arouse within the individual an innate curiosity to learn more about the science of diet and nutrition. Thus it is one's engagement with the creative process itself that stimulates the desire to learn more about the process and its underlying mechanisms. This type of learning is ecstatic learning. It is a fun sort of adventure that just kind of happens on its own.

In the process of learning about the science of diet and nutrition, the individual may discover foods that are very good for the body but that are not necessarily very appealing, though they may still be palatable. One thing to consider is that while foods of this nature may not provide immediate gratification, they may contribute to the overall process of facilitating ecstasy by cleansing the palate and/or by serving as a sort of sensorial backdrop to the more occasional, intermittent novelty of a treat.

Spacing out treats

Treats can be spaced out in a number of different ways. In the ritual of bindling, which is a day-by-day process, the most basic unit of time is the day. Therefore, the most basic way of leveraging the power of treats while bindling is by including some kind of treat every single day. For example, the individual may wish to enjoy a treat towards the end of each day, as something to look forward to throughout the day.

Another way of leveraging the power of treats while bindling is to plan on setting aside certain days—several days ahead—on which the individual plans to be especially self-indulgent. This makes it much easier to place reasonable limits on the self during the intervening days. A day that is set aside for extra self-indulgence could occur every few days, once a week, on weekends, or whenever the individual feels the need to set aside such a day.

The individual who is just starting out in the bindling process may feel the need to be extra self-indulgent every single day for a while. If that is the case, then so be it. Then, as the condition of self-mastery becomes stronger and the individual becomes more disciplined, it becomes easier—effortless, actually—to eat healthier foods for several days, knowing that a day of extra indulgence is just over the horizon.

The key to success in spacing out treats is to trust the creative process and to allow it to work itself out.

Treats can be enjoyed in solitude, as a means of direct, mystic communion with the creative process, or they can be part of one's participation in a social eating ritual.

Social eating rituals

A social eating ritual is an eating situation in which the individual may have less control over the specific types and amounts of foods that are eaten. This loss of control can be part of the pleasure of a social eating ritual, wherein the individual becomes absorbed into the social gathering and experiences the elements of surprise and spontaneity.

Important social eating rituals are always planned at least one day in advance and therefore are highly conducive to the bindling process. The most important social eating rituals are planned weeks or months in advance, and some occur on a specified day once per year. All such occasions are potential sources of leverage in the bindling process, in that they make it so much easier for the individual to place reasonable limits on the self during the days, weeks, and/or months during which the individual looks forward to participating in any such social eating ritual.

Over time the individual who bindles may become more selective about the specific social eating rituals in which the individual chooses to participate. Bindling can be thought of as a way of having an internal conversation with the self, as a means of figuring out and deciding on the specific social eating rituals in which the individual genuinely wishes to participate.

Immersive social eating rituals

From time to time, there may be a series of a few days or so—for example, while on a family vacation or while traveling to an exotic location with a friend—during which the individual may wish to become fully absorbed in the experience and simply eat all meals with the other people or person with whom the individual is sharing the vacation or the trip or whatever it may be. During an experience of this nature, sharing food with one another and eating communally for a few days may be a defining feature of the experience.

Throughout the duration of an experience of this nature, the individual may wish to refrain from using the obtained category on the bindling forms and instead, in the ritualized category, write something along the lines of,

Whatever I wish to eat of food (a) I share with [insert name(s) or collective name of other(s) present], (b) [insert name(s)] share(s) with me, and (c) [insert name(s)] and I get and eat together

— and then, as usual, write out the obtained alternate plan. In this way, the individual is able to become fully immersed in the experience. In fact, the individual's immersion and indulgence in the experience is deepened when the individual's eating is tethered to the social ritual that is occurring.

Immersive social eating rituals that continue for several days tend to allow for the highest levels of indulgence, and provide the individual with a much needed break from the everyday routines and stresses of life. Because immersive social eating rituals allow for high levels of indulgence while also providing the individual with some much needed down time and recuperation, they serve as very powerful sources of leverage in the bindling process during the days, weeks, and months leading up to such events. The excitement of looking forward to an immersive social eating ritual makes it so much easier to place reasonable limits on the self during the time leading up to it.

Other ways to bindle during a trip

When traveling alone or even while traveling with others, the individual may wish to try out other, less communal (i.e., less socially immersive) ways of bindling during the trip that still allow the individual to explore and enjoy the foods that are available in the visited destination.

For example, during a visit to a town that has several appealing restaurants, an entry in the ritualized category might be something along the lines of,

Whatever I wish to eat at a visit to a restaurant of my choice

—followed, as usual, with an obtained alternate plan. In this way, the individual is able to designate the bounds of a specific eating ritual wherein the individual gets to have fun with the process of exploring the various restaurants that are available and deciding on one to visit.

Honoring cravings

In addition to accentuating the pleasure of various types of special eating occasions, bindling provides the individual with a means of systematically honoring cravings on a regular basis, during the ordinary, day-by-day life of the individual.

The key to effectively honoring cravings is to begin to notice the difference between momentary cravings and deep cravings, and to then focus one's attention on honoring deep cravings.

Momentary cravings. Momentary cravings are generally triggered by something we see or smell. Cravings of this nature tend to fade away out of the mind within a few minutes. Momentary cravings come and go all the time, though in the individual who bindles, over time such cravings may lose their sticking power and hardly even register in the mind at all.

Deep cravings. A deep craving is rooted in the psyche, and while it may be evoked by a sensory experience, it is a desire that stays with the individual for a longer amount of time. A deep craving is a very specific desire for a particular food item that returns to the mind again and again. So long as the individual has access to this specific food item and genuinely wishes to introduce it into the body, the individual honors the craving by bindling the item to be enjoyed the following day.

A certain craving may appear in the psyche again and again, maybe even for several days in a row. In this case, the task of the individual is simply to continue to honor the craving until its needs have been satisfied, and to fully enjoy its presence during the time in which it is requesting the attention of the individual.

As the individual gets into the bindling process, feelings of enjoyment and excitement about the process and about the transformations that are occurring in the life of the individual may eliminate many of the individual's cravings for excess food. Such is the nature of becoming caught up in a creative process.

At the same time, the process of bindling ensures that the individual is always eating adequate amounts of food. Unlike a willy nilly eating process, in which the individual may go back and forth between phases of eating too much and phases of eating too little,

129

bindling brings into the life of the individual an overarching, non-ruminative moderation, and an underlying quality of balance.

Exploring the Ecstasy of Eating

Bindling is a technique of ecstasy that accentuates the pleasures of eating by heightening the individual's awareness of the ongoing eating process. As this process evolves, the individual gets to have fun and experiment with various approaches to the eating process, to discover ways of optimizing its ecstatic quality.

Cooking is a way of exploring various types of food items and becoming intimately familiar with the unique nuances of various items. Also, the process of cooking facilitates the individual entering into the psychospiritual condition of paradoxical mindful mindlessness, which heightens the individual's ability to perceive and appreciate the most subtle of nuances.

Preparing and/or cooking some or most of one's own meals at home is also a way of heightening the pleasure of a meal prepared by someone else, or an occasional meal enjoyed at a restaurant.

The individual may wish to experiment with eating extremely simple meals, as a way of becoming intimately familiar with the unique nuances of specific foods and combinations of foods. Sometimes, when a specific food or combination of foods is eaten repeatedly over several consecutive days, the individual begins to experience it on deeper levels and to appreciate it in new ways. It's sort of like with a really great album, in the sense that it may take a few listens before the beauty and magic of it really begin to sink in.

The individual may wish to experiment with various ways of making the eating process special and sacred every day. For example, it can be very nice to set aside some time towards the end of the day for a dinner ritual, during which food is prepared and then enjoyed on nice dishes. A dinner ritual facilitates mystic communion with the creative process, and can be enjoyed in solitude or in communion with others.

The individual may wish to experiment with various factors that contribute to the atmosphere of the space in which a dinner ritual is experienced. For example, a meal can be enjoyed in silence, with gentle conversation, while listening to music or an audiobook, or while watching a documentary or a television program. Also, dimming the lights and/or using candles is a way to create sacred space for an evening meal.

During the process of introducing any type of food into the body, whether liquid or solid, there are various details and nuances that are available to be noticed and appreciated. There is

the way a food item looks, the way it smells,

the way it feels on the fingers when it is touched or broken apart, the texture, the temperature, the sounds,

the way it feels to take hold of the food and to carry it to the mouth,

the feeling of the food on the lips,

the sensations on the teeth and tongue, on all the various surfaces inside the mouth,

the feeling of the liquid or the morsel of food inside the mouth,

the chemical reactions that occur on the tongue, the intricate details of the flavors, the texture, the temperature, the sounds,

the feeling of chewing the food, the repeated motion of the jaw,

swallowing the food, the feeling of the food in the throat, in the digestive tract,

the feeling of the food as it moves through the body,

any changes in temperature inside the body,

changes in the way a food item tastes and is experienced across repeated bites,

the beauty of the empty bowl or plate after a meal,

the lingering feeling of a meal being absorbed into the body,

upon awakening the next day, how the body feels after having eaten certain types of foods on the previous day . .

. the individual's energy level, the feeling in the brain and in various parts of the body,

changes in the way a food item tastes and is experienced when it is eaten repeatedly across a series of consecutive days,

and feelings of pleasure that occur when the undigested remains of various types of food and of various combinations of food are excreted from the body.

The sensuality of the eating experience is something to experiment with and explore, not something that has to be done in a certain way. Approaching the process in a spirit of experimentation and play is part of the pleasure of the process.

One way of appreciating the full details and nuances that are available is to chew a morsel of food to its full, absolute completion, to pause, and to then have another bite. It feels good to notice all of the various sensations that occur at each point along this process, and to observe the timing of the process and the feelings of anticipation.

At the same time, the individual may wish to experiment with just being boring about the eating process and not focusing so meticulously on being so appreciative of every last detail.

The Primacy of Effortlessness

Effortlessness is the most basic key to a successful and satisfying bindling process. If the process ever begins to feel too complicated or burdensome, the most important task of the individual is to find a way to simplify the process and bring it back to its effortless quality.

Effortlessness during initiation

Effortlessness is especially important during the initial phase during which the individual is just starting out with the bindling process. All creative processes at least initially involve some discomfort as the psyche begins to engage itself with anything that is new or that involves change.

Getting started with bindling is similar to the process of priming a pump: The process begins with an initial challenge of bringing liquid into the pump, but then once it starts to flow, the process takes over and continues on its own, effortlessly.

Bindling is initiated through the Three-Day Initiation Cycle, yet on a deeper, emotional level, the initiation process may take a little longer. During this initial phase of getting used to a new process and a new type of sacred space in one's life, the most important thing is for the individual to find ways of soothing the self, ways to be kind and gentle with the self as it transitions into a new process. An initial phase of discomfort occurs at the beginning of almost any creative process that is truly gratifying.

134

Experiencing the discomfort and figuring out the best ways to soothe the self is an important learning process that eventually becomes embedded into the ongoing bindling process, and into the individual's ongoing way of being in the world.

Effortlessness ongoing

As the bindling process evolves, the individual continues to discover new ways to simplify the process and to keep it as effortless as is possible. Effortlessness is paradoxical, and so the more the individual keeps the bindling process effortless, the more the individual actually gets into it.

When the individual keeps the bindling process as effortless as is possible, the process itself takes over and refines itself, seemingly of its own accord.

As the bindling process refines itself and the individual's desired outcome begins to materialize, the task of the individual is simply to maintain stillness within the self. Success in bindling is achieved not by pushing or pulling of the self, but rather by continually remaining in one's comfort zone, and allowing the refinements and transitions that occur to be so gradual that they are nearly imperceptible to the individual. This paradoxical approach gives the creative process the space it needs to take over and create something miraculous in the life of the individual.

When the individual maintains a stance of stillness within the self, this allows the individual to become a channel through which the innate movement of the creative process itself becomes manifested.

The creative process is continually in motion. Movement is the most basic, universal quality of the creative process. We have yet to discover a single location in the universe where anything remains stationary. This is as true for entire galaxies as it is for subatomic particles.

The creative process, our source, is doing plenty of moving on its own. Our task is simply to align ourselves, via ritual, such that the creative process delivers to us the specific outcomes we desire.

The Bindle

Each day of life is a brand new journey, and to bindle is to fully experience it in this way. The individual's daily completion of the daily bindling ritual invokes within the psyche a very deep sense of sacredness, and of reverence for the journey to come.

Self-Mastery

Bindling is a technique of ecstasy wherein the individual effortlessly releases excess weight and permanently maintains desired bodily form simply by creating the powerful psychospiritual condition of self-mastery.

By deliberately creating the condition of self-mastery, the individual bypasses a surface-level focus on food content and goes directly to the heart of the matter within the deeper levels of the psyche.

The psychospiritual condition of self-mastery is absolutely the most powerful and effective ingredient in the effortless releasing of excess weight and the permanent maintenance of desired bodily form.

The condition of self-mastery operates within the deeper levels of the psyche and produces profound, pervasive ripple effects in the life of the individual that go far beyond the original desired outcome. Self-mastery empowers the individual to get and do all things the individual wishes to get and do. The psychospiritual condition of self-mastery is the fountainhead of all achievements in life.

Bindling is an especially powerful way of producing the condition of self-mastery because of the fact that the condition is produced within the domain of diet. Diet is the most basic biological process required for the survival of the organism over which the individual is able to deliberately exert choice.

There are so many choices and options available to the individual in the domain of diet, a domain that is inextricably linked to the basic survival of the individual as a living organism.

By bindling, the individual is able to make deliberate choices and to follow through with those choices in this reasonably challenging domain, and to thereby enter into the immensely powerful condition of self-mastery.

The individual who bindles creates the condition of self-mastery not by coming up with the perfect combination of foods, but rather, simply, by following through with whatever it is that was planned the day before, knowing that the individual had full freedom to put whatever was desired (of available foods) on the menu for the day.

As the condition of self-mastery gains strength and momentum, the bindling process refines itself and the desired outcome begins to materialize. This is something that happens on its own; it is an occurrence that is witnessed by the individual.

The individual simply focuses on the innately ecstatic process of creating the condition of self-mastery in a relaxed, effortless manner. No direct pressure is placed on the self to release the excess weight and maintain the desired bodily form. The creative process takes care of this.

The individual who bindles develops a deep, profound, unflinching discipline that is paradoxically effortless because it is motivated by ecstasy and is energized by ecstasy on an ongoing basis.

Actions that are ecstatic feel as if they are happening on their own, and require no pushing or pulling of the self. They are like blinking, taking a deep breath, or turning in one's sleep—they just kind of happen on their own.

The key to facilitating this sort of paradoxically effortless, ecstatic discipline in the bindling process is to always keep the bar ridiculously low, to always make sure it is well within the comfort zone of the individual to set a particular plan and follow through with it. This is all that is required of the individual. The rest is taken care of by the creative process.

Ownership of Self

Deliberate creation of the powerful psychospiritual condition of self-mastery opens up the life of the individual to all of the gifts and possibilities of life. To deliberately create the condition of self-mastery is to deliberately claim ownership of self, and to thereby gain access to all of the gifts and possibilities of life, to all of the very best that life has to offer.

The individual who claims ownership of self embraces full ownership of the executive functioning of the psyche, becomes the protagonist in the individual's own life, and thereby gains access to all of the very best that life has to offer.

The self is the final frontier. To claim ownership of self is to fully embrace the idea that I am an adult, and that I accept responsibility for the care, nourishment, and satisfaction of the self. Making this claim within the psyche is the first step in the fulfillment of one's potential as a human being.

Wonderful as it is to claim ownership of self and to thereby gain access to all of the very best that life has to offer, we may resist doing so due to the simple fact that we are womb-creatures, and as such, our very origin is dependency.

Prior to our claiming ownership of self, our natural inclination is to behave like helpless infants, like baby birds with our beaks up in the air, waiting for mother to bring us a worm. Even after we are fully developed physically and are fully capable of providing for ourselves, we continue to look to other people and to institutions to recreate for us the womb of origin, to recreate for us the place where all our needs are met in warmth and dark silence.

Our strivings to return to the womb or to discover a surrogate womb created for us by someone else never actually lead us into a condition of having our needs met. Ultimately such strivings only end up bringing us misery.

At the end of the day, the bottom line is that seeking out a condition of dependency prevents us from claiming ownership of self and thereby gaining access to all of the very best that life has to offer.

So it is up to the individual then to decide: Do I want to keep looking for someone or something else to keep changing my diaper for me, or do I want to claim ownership of self and thereby gain access to all of the very best that life has to offer?

The individual who resists claiming ownership of self and who continues to live in ambivalence about making this claim within the psyche may instead seek to dominate others and/or to be dominated by them.

Ultimately what happens when an otherwise mature adult refuses to claim ownership of self is that this individual becomes a supporting character in someone or something else's story, and becomes subject to the whims of that person's or institution's narrative.

Claiming ownership of self is not an act against the womb of origin. Rather, it is a paradoxical process that works in deep cooperation with our innate and irrevocable nature as womb-creatures. To claim ownership of self is to mature beyond the womb of origin, to mature past passivity and dependency, by recreating for oneself in adulthood the nurturing conditions of the womb, i.e., by caring for oneself and tending to one's needs on a continual, ongoing basis.

To claim ownership of self in this paradoxical way, in deep cooperation with our innate and irrevocable nature as womb-creatures, grants us the highest level of access to all of the very best that life has to offer. This highest level of access is something

145

that cannot be bestowed on a person by someone else; it is something that can only be claimed by the individual who wishes to experience this highest level of access.

Bindling facilitates the claiming of ownership of self in this paradoxical way, in deep cooperation with our innate and irrevocable nature as womb-creatures. Bindling provides the individual with a way of maturing beyond the womb of origin and simultaneously recreating for oneself the nurturing conditions of the womb in adulthood.

The individual who bindles claims ownership of self by taking good care of the self on an ongoing basis, and because this occurs in the foundational domain of diet—the most basic biological process over which the individual is able to deliberately exert choice—the claiming of and caring for the self becomes a theme that becomes deeply embedded into all aspects of the life of the individual.

This process has a ripple effect wherein the eyes of the individual begin to be opened up to the multitude of opportunities that are out there and available to whoever wishes to claim them, but which normally go unnoticed and untapped. The individual who claims ownership of self experiences an alteration of consciousness wherein the individual develops a keen capacity for perceiving exactly how to access all of the very best and the very finest that life has to offer.

When the individual bindles, the individual enters into an optimal alignment or positioning of the self, an alignment that facilitates the individual receiving a desired outcome delivered to the self by the creative process. Simply being in this position leads the individual to naturally begin to discover other positions and alignments whereby all other desired outcomes can be effortlessly delivered to the individual by the creative process.

The global infrastructures and systems of our world today have left many of us feeling helpless and unsure about how to achieve our goals and to get what we want out of life. At the moment of greatest abundance and opportunity, many of us are actually at a complete loss about what to do next.

The first step in figuring out how to get what we want from the systems that surround us is to claim ownership of the most basic system over which we have dominion—the body—and to then simply allow the ripple effects to occur.

When we place ourselves into the powerful psychospiritual condition of self-mastery and thereby claim ownership of self, our ways of perceiving and of being in the world become transformed in their entirety. We will explore exactly how this happens in greater detail in the next chapter, Transformation of Self.

Self-Mastery and Others

Creating for oneself the powerful psychospiritual condition of self-mastery and thereby claiming ownership of self is not a good thing or a bad thing; it is neither right nor wrong. Rather, self-mastery is simply a resource, a source of power that is available to the individual who wishes to claim it. The individual who deliberately creates the condition of self-mastery is not better than others; rather, this person is simply more powerful.

Therefore, there is never any reason to preach to others about why the individual feels that others "should" place themselves into this condition. To fully claim ownership of self is to keep one's focus on oneself and to not try to manage the lives of others.

In fact, the individual who bindles can keep the bindling process completely invisible to others, and need not ever explain it to others unless there is an innate desire to do so.

When the individual is bindling, another person may spontaneously offer a food item to the individual. There are various ways in which the individual may respond to a food offering and maintain respect for both the self and the other.

The individual may wish to accept the food offering and express an intention to enjoy the item later. This can either be explained (e.g., "I have something else to eat") or left unexplained.

The individual may wish to graciously say no thank you to the food offering. This can either be explained (e.g., "I have something else to eat") or left unexplained.

If the individual does like to accept spontaneous food offerings and save them for an upcoming day (provided it's not something that will melt or spoil), it's a good idea to keep a plastic zipper storage bag tucked away. This way, an item that is received can be saved and bindled for enjoyment on a subsequent day.

Self-Mastery Egress

Bindling is a technique of ecstasy, and as such, it is never something that "should" be done. Bindling rather is simply a potential source of power and a great starting point for living one's life to its fullest potential. The process creates deep levels of ecstasy and transforms the life of the individual in its entirety, but it is never something that has to be done.

Therefore, if for whatever reason the individual ever goes through a self-mastery egress prior to having planned to do so, this need only be viewed as a development in one's innate and irrevocable relationship with the creative process.

Self-mastery creates a specific type of sacred space in the life of the individual, but it is important to recognize first and foremost that the individual is innately sacred, i.e., the individual is an innately sacred manifestation of the creative process— regardless of whether or not the individual ever enters and/or egresses any type of sacred space.

The sacred space of self-mastery is a setting in which the innately sacred and divine individual is facilitated in receiving desired outcomes. It would be a blasphemy to ever infer from this that the sacred space confers upon the individual the individual's innate and irrevocable sacredness and divinity.

The individual is sacred and divine, because the individual is.

I am that I am.

The individual is innately divine, for the individual is a manifestation of the creative process. This is something that cannot ever be altered or changed. It is as innate and irrevocable as the universe itself, as the creative process itself.

Therefore, if the individual ever goes through a self-mastery egress prior to having planned to do so, there really are no justifiable grounds for judging, condemning, or getting down on oneself in any way. In a situation of this nature, the innately sacred and divine individual has simply stepped outside the bounds of a particular type of sacred space and can, as soon as is desired, enter into that sacred space again through the Three-Day Initiation Cycle.

If the individual ever goes through a self-mastery egress prior to having planned to do so, the individual need only accept what has happened.

The individual may wish to consider possible meanings of the egress, possible reasons why it occurred, in a spirit of curious introspection.

Before entering into the sacred space of self-mastery again through the Three-Day Initiation Cycle, the individual may wish to simply meditate on the beauty of the concept of effortlessness, of emptiness, of the void . . . to step back fully . . . . . . and to then allow the deeper levels of the psyche to present to the mind new ways of allowing the quality of effortlessness to become manifested throughout the entirety of one's ongoing bindling process.

The individual may go through a premature self-mastery egress several times, over and over again. If this is what happens, so be it. It need only be accepted and, if anything, used as material for curious introspection. It is never a reason for allowing even a scrap of self-condemnation.

Everything that we experience can be reframed and redirected into the deepening of our ecstatic relationship with the creative process. Everything can be channelized into helping us to evolve, to explore, and to engage ourselves with the creative process as it is manifested inside us, around us, and in every last corner of the universe in its entirety.

Transformation of Self

Bindling is a technique of ecstasy wherein the individual focuses simply on creating the powerful psychospiritual condition of self-mastery, and thereby turns over the task of effortlessly releasing excess weight and permanently maintaining desired bodily form to the creative process as it is manifested in the deeper levels of the psyche.

Deliberate creation of the psychospiritual condition of self-mastery is the single most important ingredient in the process of effortlessly releasing excess weight and permanently maintaining desired bodily form. When the individual deliberately creates the psychospiritual condition of self-mastery via the bindling ritual, the individual simultaneously activates within the deeper levels of the psyche a deeper, underlying process wherein the self becomes transformed in its entirety.

This deeper, underlying transformation of self process is carried out not through the conscious deliberation of the individual; rather, it is carried out by the creative process as it is manifested in the deeper levels of the psyche. The individual simply witnesses this process as it unfolds.

This deeper, underlying transformation of self process is inextricably linked to the condition of self-mastery in that it is the creation of the condition of self-mastery that activates the transformation of self process and sets it into motion. The vast bulk of the process, however, is carried out not through the conscious deliberation of the individual but rather through the deeper workings of the creative process.

In a sense, then, deliberate creation of the condition of self-mastery via the bindling ritual is merely a gesture. To place oneself into the condition of self-mastery is like turning on a switch that activates the circuitry of a much larger process, the majority of which is outside the direct, conscious influence of the individual. The switch simply serves to activate the process.

The transformation of self process becomes activated immediately in the very moment in which the individual enters into the condition of self-mastery, and the transformation of self process deepens and becomes more pervasive the longer the individual remains in the condition of self-mastery.

Although the transformation of self process is inextricably linked to the condition of self-mastery that activates it, at the same time the transformation of self process is less distinct and more pervasive than the condition of self-mastery. Therefore, the transformation of self process continues regardless of egresses from the condition of self-mastery, provided the individual reenters the condition of self-mastery.

In fact, egresses from and reentries into the condition of self-mastery may in some cases even deepen the transformation of self process. This can occur even when there is a gap of time (regardless of its duration) between an egress and a reentry into the condition of self-mastery.

Formation of the Charge

The transformation of self process becomes activated immediately in the very moment in which the individual enters into the condition of self-mastery. From that point on, the full unfolding of the transformation of self process revolves around the gradual, ongoing formation of a powerful charge between the individual and the desired outcome, i.e., between the individual and the individual's desired bodily form.

This powerful charge between the individual and the desired outcome forms and gains strength as a function of the individual desiring the outcome while the psyche is in the psychospiritual condition of self-mastery. It is the co-occurrence of these two ingredients, (a) self-mastery and (b) desiring the outcome, that facilitates the formation and strengthening of the powerful charge between the individual and the desired outcome.

As the individual's desire for the outcome circulates fully within the psyche while the psyche is in the powerful psychospiritual condition of self-mastery, this powerful charge between the individual and the desired outcome becomes stronger and stronger, and the individual thereby enters into the condition of inevitability, the condition in which the individual's desired bodily form becomes inevitable and materializes.

At the same time, while this powerful charge between the individual and the desired outcome forms within the psyche and increases in strength, the creative process responds to the presence of this charge and carries out a deep and comprehensive rearranging and reconfiguring of the entire psyche and life of the individual — all in surround of the powerful charge between the individual and the individual's desired bodily form.

A New Arrangement of Self

The transformation of self process that is carried out by the creative process in surround of the powerful charge between the individual and the individual's desired bodily form is the deepest and the most pervasive transformation of self that is possible to be experienced because of the fact that it is activated by means of diet, the most basic biological process required for the survival of the organism over which the individual is able to deliberately exert choice.

This deep and comprehensive transformation of self process reaches deeply into the totality of the being of the individual, into the oneness that is spirit and flesh. It reaches deeply into all aspects of the psyche and the life of the individual, such that the original desired outcome, the individual's desired bodily form, comes to be just one of its numerous manifestations.

Transformation of self is a transpersonal experience that brings the individual into the deepest and most direct communion with the divine presence that interconnects and interpenetrates all that is. It is the deepest and the most mysterious of all creative processes, and it carries the individual into the utmost realms of the divine, the infinite, the universal.

Within the psyche, the transformation of self process is guided by the place of dreaming, which is a manifestation of the creative process within the self. As the transformation of self process proceeds, the place of dreaming formulates a new arrangement of self in surround of the powerful charge between the individual and the individual's desired bodily form.

Because the transformation of self process is guided by the place of dreaming, it results in a reconfiguration of the psyche and the life of the individual that is far more satisfying than what the individual could have ever achieved through conscious deliberation alone.

Riding Out the Transformation

To activate the transformation of self process and allow it to unfold in one's life is to allow a mysterious process to become initiated deep within the psyche, the outcome of which is something entirely new and resplendent. In the transformation of self process, everything gets shifted around for the better in the life of the individual, and the individual enters into a whole new life, a whole new way of being in the world.

In any type of transformation, and especially in a transformation of this depth and magnitude, it is inevitable that the individual who goes through the transformation process will encounter uncomfortable feelings as the process proceeds. Feelings of discomfort and dysphoria are inevitable whenever the psyche experiences change, and the most important aspect of coping with such emotions is simply to accept that they are inevitable when transformation occurs.

At the same time, when dysphoric emotions arise during the transformation of self process, this provides the individual with an opportunity to begin to discover and develop new ways of soothing the self and new ways of coping with discomfort—that is, other than willy nilly eating of excess food.

For example, the individual may experience soothing through participation in a hobby, or by visiting with a friend, or through the immense healing power of humor. The most effective of all self-soothing, coping strategies is to deepen one's level of engagement with the creative process. We will explore this topic in greater detail in the Desired Outcome chapter.

The key to successfully riding out any and all uncomfortable emotions that may arise during the transformation of self process is to approach one's emotional life in the same way that a nurturing parent attends to the emotions of a newborn child.

This involves recognizing that no emotion is ever right or wrong, being gentle with oneself continually, and, when dysphoric emotions arise, figuring out the best possible ways to respond to them and to soothe the self.

160

Then, as the individual develops new strategies for coping with uncomfortable emotions during the transformation of self process, these new coping strategies evolve into new patterns of coping that become seamlessly embedded into the transformed self, i.e., they become naturally integrated into the individual's whole new way of being in the world.

The transformation of self process does arouse feelings of discomfort, and it may even feel scary at times, yet these emotions are actually part of what make the transformation of self process the exciting adventure that it is. Reasonable levels of fear and discomfort occur at the beginning of all true adventures.

Ripple Effects of the Transformation

The transformation of self process is not a process of transformation from bad to good, or from unholy to holy. Rather, it is a process of transformation from less powerful to more powerful, and from less ecstatic to more ecstatic.

The individual is a manifestation of the creative process, and as such, the individual is innately and irrevocably holy and divine. In the transformation of self process, the innately and irrevocably holy and divine individual simply goes through a developmental, evolutionary process of transformation that facilitates the individual receiving a specific desired outcome, getting more out of life, falling in love with the void, and experiencing the most extraordinary levels of ecstasy that are possible to be experienced.

The individual is innately and irrevocably holy and divine before, during, and after the transformation of self process. The transformation of self process simply makes life better for the individual. It delivers to the individual the desired outcome and simultaneously reconfigures the psyche in such a way that other desired outcomes and transformations become easily delivered to the self.

Therefore, regardless of whatever various life transformations the individual may wish to experience, and regardless of whatever specific outcomes the individual may wish to have delivered to the self, participation in the bindling ritual to create the condition of self-mastery and thereby activate the transformation of self process is by far the most powerful and effective way to initiate the effortless occurrence of all such desired transformations and outcomes.

It Is Simply a Process

The transformation of self process that is activated when the individual enters the condition of self-mastery via the bindling ritual is truly the deepest and the most magical and mysterious of all creative processes. At the same time, it is simply a process, and it need only be activated to be experienced.

The transformation of self process is available to all, such that any person who chooses to activate it will experience its unfolding. Any person who enters into the condition of self-mastery via the bindling ritual and then allows desire for the outcome to circulate throughout the psyche while the psyche remains in the condition of self-mastery will experience and witness the full unfolding of the transformation of self process.

Twin Key Processes

The two ongoing processes of (a) bindling and (b) desiring the outcome are the two only domains in which it is necessary and useful for the individual to deliberately exert conscious influence over the ongoing transformation of self process. Focusing one's attention simply on these twin key processes allows one's energy to remain focused simply on the formation of the powerful charge that is at the center of the transformation of self process.

As the individual focuses simply on bindling and desiring the outcome, this charge becomes stronger and stronger, and the creative process correspondingly responds to the presence and the strengthening of this charge by carrying out the transformation of self process in its mysterious entirety, all in surround of the powerful charge between the individual and the desired outcome.

Desiring with confidence

Of the twin key processes of bindling and desiring the outcome, bindling is the basic, foundational task that serves the function of creating the psychospiritual condition of self-mastery and thereby initiating the activation of the ongoing transformation of self process.

The other of the twin key processes, desiring the outcome, is a less distinct, less ritualized process that simply involves the circulation of desire for the outcome within the psyche while the psyche is in the condition of self-mastery.

While desiring the outcome is a less distinct, less ritualized process in comparison to the process of bindling, at the same time it is an essential ingredient in the transformation of self process. It is through the process of desiring the outcome while the psyche is in the condition of self-mastery that the powerful charge that is at the center of the entire transformation of self process forms.

Participation in the ritual of bindling is important in that it provides the individual with the ability to begin to desire the outcome with confidence. Because the individual is participating in the bindling ritual, the individual knows that the psyche has now become a crucible of transformation in which the individual's desire for the outcome is able to circulate freely and to thereby form the powerful charge between the individual and the desired outcome that is at the center of the transformation of self process.

Knowing that the psyche has now become a crucible of transformation as a function of one's participation in the bindling ritual provides the individual with the freedom to fully and deliberately desire the outcome, and to fully and deliberately release oneself into the ongoing desiring process.

Before the individual began the process of bindling, desiring the outcome of releasing excess weight and permanently maintaining desired bodily form may have created feelings of dysphoria and ambivalence. Feelings of desire for the outcome

164

may have been offset by feelings of helplessness about how to go about bringing the desired outcome into material reality.

In fact, the individual may have felt so many dysphoric emotions while desiring or attempting to desire the outcome, that the individual may have developed ways to avoid desiring the outcome altogether, in order to avoid the dysphoric emotions evoked by the desiring process.

Once the individual begins to bindle, it then becomes safe for the individual to begin to desire the outcome with full confidence that the outcome is now in the process of being delivered to the self, i.e., that the psyche has now become a crucible of transformation wherein the desired outcome is beginning to materialize.

Once the individual understands that the psyche has now become a crucible of transformation on account of the individual's participation in the bindling ritual, the individual can then actually begin to have fun with the process of desiring the outcome.

The individual can then begin to desire the outcome with excitement and anticipation, with the understanding that allowing desire for the outcome to circulate fully within the psyche while the psyche is in the condition of self-mastery is actually essential for the formation of the powerful charge that is at the center of the entire transformation of self process.

In the next chapter, Condition of Inevitability, we will explore ways in which the individual is able to deliberately deepen the process of desiring the outcome so as to strengthen the powerful charge that is at the center of the transformation of self process — and thereby to accelerate one's entry into the condition of inevitability.

Ecstasy and desire

Underlying the twin key processes of bindling and desiring the outcome are the basic psychospiritual processes of ecstasy and desire. Specifically, ecstasy is the basic psychospiritual process underlying bindling, and desire is the basic psychospiritual process underlying desiring the outcome.

Ecstasy underlies bindling in that bindling is a technique of ecstasy that produces multiple levels of ecstasy that reinforce and energize the ongoing bindling process.

Desire underlies desiring the outcome in that desiring the outcome is an outcome-specific expression of one's innate, underlying desiring process.

Therefore, to focus one's energy and attention simply on the twin key processes of bindling and desiring the outcome is to dwell entirely in ecstasy and desire. Dwelling entirely in ecstasy and desire in this way keeps the individual completely out of the way of the creative process, and gives the creative process the space it needs to carry out the full transformation of self.

At the same time, dwelling entirely in ecstasy and desire by focusing simply on bindling and desiring the outcome facilitates the full ongoing circulation of ecstasy and desire within the psyche, which provides the creative process with the energizing fuel it needs on an ongoing basis to carry out the full transformation of self.

Both the transformation of self process and the processes of ecstasy and desire that energize the transformation of self process are manifestations of the divine, i.e., they are manifestations of the creative process within the self.

Therefore, to dwell entirely in ecstasy and desire by focusing simply on bindling and desiring the outcome is to dwell entirely in the divine, and to bring oneself into perfect alignment with the creative process. Dwelling entirely in ecstasy and desire in this way gives the creative process both the space it needs and the energizing fuel that it needs on an ongoing basis to carry out the transformation of self in its mysterious entirety.

Releasing shame and should

When the individual does not allow ecstasy and desire to circulate throughout the psyche and instead blocks the innate flowing of ecstasy and desire, this may be due to the introduction of shame and/or should into the psyche. Shame is feeling badly about the self and about the processes of ecstasy and desire within the self, and "should" is shorthand for doing something out of obligation only, rather than out of an innate desire to do the thing.

If the individual has developed a pattern of recycling shame and should within the psyche, yet wishes to allow the transformation of self process to occur, then first it is up to the individual to release shame and should so that ecstasy and desire are able to circulate freely within the psyche and to thereby energize the full unfolding of the transformation of self process.

Releasing shame and should does not preclude the individual from being conscientious about the consequences of the individual's behavior, or from being considerate of the well-being of persons and following through with commitments. What releasing shame and should entails is refraining from feeling badly about the self and about the processes of ecstasy and desire within the self, and honoring the individual's innate desiring process by choosing behaviors in which the individual innately desires to participate.

Certainly it is good for the individual to feel remorse when the individual has caused any type of harm to a person. This though is very different from feeling shame about the self and about the processes of ecstasy and desire within the self.

Certainly it is good for the individual to follow through with commitments the individual has made with others. This though is very different from living in should and systematically ignoring on an ongoing basis the innate desires of the self.

Whereas shame and should are superimposed on the psyche, ecstasy and desire are innate manifestations of the creative process within the psyche of the individual.

Shame and should are conducive with stuckness and retention of excess weight.

Ecstasy and desire are conducive with movement, and with the effortless releasing of excess weight and the permanent maintenance of desired bodily form.

The more the individual has recycled shame and should in the past, the more likely it is that the individual will be frightened to allow ecstasy and desire to circulate fully within the psyche. In an extreme case the individual may have even gotten to the point of demonizing ecstasy and desire altogether, i.e., demonizing the creative process itself as it is manifested within the psyche of the individual.

The individual who has dieted or considered dieting in the past is likely to have an acute familiarity with shame in particular. This may have involved shame about the individual's body, shame about self-perceived failures in dieting, and shame about having ever felt the need to diet at all.

Shame may be so pervasive in an individual or in a society as a whole that persons may become acclimated to it, pass it down from one generation to the next, and treat it as though it is more innate to the self than the processes of ecstasy and desire that it blocks and suffocates.

This widespread acclimation to shame may lead an individual to the erroneous belief that shame can be used as a motivator for an effective dieting process. Shame, in fact, is conducive with stuckness and the retention of excess weight, and with sabotaging of the dieting process. A psyche that lives in shame feels undeserving of the self-care that is embodied in the process of providing to the self a carefully selected diet.

169

Ultimately a psyche that is ruled by shame will sabotage all shame-motivated goals. To the individual who has become acclimated to shame, it may seem as if the shame is innate to the psyche, but a brief review of one's personal history is all that is required to discover that shame in fact is learned, i.e., that it is superimposed on the psyche. If this superimposed shame then is allowed to expand and to achieve dominion over the psyche, it then becomes a tyrant that keeps the individual feeling badly about the self and that blocks the innate circulation of ecstasy and desire within the psyche.

When a psyche is ruled by shame, the individual does not feel deserving of any desired outcome. In fact, the shame-ruled psyche actually is not capable of genuinely desiring anything. When shame is in charge, the individual comes to be so out of touch with the blocked processes of ecstasy and desire that the individual never actually gets to truly desire any specific goal or outcome.

What the psyche begins to do instead is to come up with goals that are not things or experiences that are genuinely desired, but rather are accomplishments that the individual erroneously believes will make the shame go away.

This is where should comes into the picture. Eventually everything the shame-ruled self does is done out of a dreary sense of obligation, beneath which lies an erroneous fantasy that once enough shame-motivated goals have been met, at long last the sense of shame will finally go away once and for all.

When a shame-ruled individual accomplishes a goal, the shame may abate for a brief moment, but soon thereafter, as long

170

as shame remains boss, feelings of shame resurface and the self comes up with new goals that it hopes will finally cause the shame to go away for good, once and for all.

The thing is, this never works. When shame is the reason for the season, the reason for achieving the goal, then shame is reinforced, shame wins and gets even more power than it had before.

The only way to get rid of shame and should from the psyche is to stop working so hard at getting rid of them.

We release shame and should, simply, by releasing them. It is very easy to do this once we come to the realization that shame and should are not innate, that they are superimposed on the psyche.

As we release shame and should, we are able then to breathe in and take in the abundance of life itself . . . . As we release shame and should, we are able then to relax and channelize our energy into honoring the innate flowing of the creative process within the self, as it is manifested in the innate flowing processes of ecstasy and desire.

We release shame and should not because they are shameful or because they should not be felt. Rather, we release them because they are ineffective, because they keep the psyche blocked and prevent the individual from receiving desired things and experiences.

Shame and should don't go away when we attack them, when we shame them, or when we insist that we "should" release them. Putting the pressure on just gives shame and should more power. The only real, effective solution is, simply, to release shame and should, to release the grip and let go of them completely. Then, as the innate processes of ecstasy and desire begin to flow again and to circulate fully within the psyche, we then get to have fun with these processes and to fully honor and facilitate them.

The silver lining for the individual who has spent years recycling shame and should is that all the mental energy that used to go into recycling shame and should can now be redirected into a superb bindling process. The person who has recycled shame and should in the psyche is likely to have simultaneously developed expertise in limits and structure, which—once the shame and should have been released—are essential to a creative process such as bindling.

A deliberate act of courage

The individual may understand the value of releasing shame and should, but may resist doing so simply because the individual has become accustomed to shame and should and feels at home with them, unsatisfying as they may be.

Shame and should instill in the individual a feeling of being undeserving of the good things in life, and a very deep fear of honoring ecstasy and desire. To the individual who has spent years dwelling in this feeling of being undeserving while at the same time demonizing ecstasy and desire, ecstasy and desire may come to be perceived as enemies or intruders from within the

172

psyche—and no perceived enemy is resisted with such furor as a perceived enemy from within.

The path to liberation opens up once the individual arrives at the realization that it is in fact shame and should that are the real intruders that have been superimposed on the psyche.

It is also possible that the individual may resist releasing shame and should as a way of resisting the full unfolding of the transformation of self process, i.e., to prevent ecstasy and desire from circulating within the psyche and thereby prevent ecstasy and desire from facilitating the full unfolding of the transformation of self process.

The psyche always resists change, even when it is in its best interest. The transformation of self process is a complete upheaval of one's life that facilitates a whole new life and a whole new way of being in the world. It is only natural for the psyche to resist a change of such depth and comprehensive magnitude.

For the individual who encounters such resistance, the deliberate decision to release shame and should and to fully honor and facilitate ecstasy and desire is a deliberate act of courage.

The transformed self

One important outcome of the transformation of self process is that the fundamental structure of the psyche becomes transformed such that the innate processes of ecstasy and desire become facilitated in circulating freely throughout the psyche on a continual, ongoing basis. In other words, the full ongoing circulation of ecstasy and desire throughout the psyche becomes seamlessly embedded into the basic, fundamental structure of the psyche.

This seamless embedding of channels within the psyche wherein ecstasy and desire are able to flow on a continual, ongoing basis is inevitable given that the transformation of self process itself is activated, facilitated, and energized by the processes of ecstasy and desire.

This seamless embedding of the flowing of ecstasy and desire within the transformed self is both a return to an original condition and a development of something new: The transformed self becomes atoned to its original condition, in which the innate, divine processes of ecstasy and desire are able to circulate freely throughout the psyche, and at the same time, the transformed self experiences an advanced level of psychospiritual power through which ecstasy and desire may now be channelized for the purpose of effortlessly materializing various desired transformations and outcomes.

Condition of Inevitability

The transformation of self process that is activated by the individual's participation in the ritual of bindling centers around the formation of a powerful charge between the individual and the desired outcome.

This powerful charge between the individual and the desired outcome forms as the individual's desire to effortlessly release excess weight and permanently maintain desired bodily form circulates freely throughout the psyche while the psyche is in the powerful psychospiritual condition of self-mastery.

As desire for the outcome continues to circulate throughout the psyche on an ongoing basis, the powerful charge between the individual and the desired outcome becomes stronger and stronger, and the individual thereby enters into the condition of inevitability, the condition in which the desired outcome becomes inevitable and materializes.

The individual who bindles is able to desire the outcome with confidence, because the individual who bindles understands that the psyche has now become a crucible of transformation in which the ongoing process of desiring the outcome contributes to the strengthening of the powerful charge wherein the individual enters into the condition of inevitability.

In fact, once the psyche has become a crucible of transformation via the individual's participation in the bindling ritual, the ongoing process of desiring the outcome becomes an essential activating ingredient in the ongoing process of strengthening the powerful charge between the individual and the desired outcome, wherein the desired outcome becomes inevitable and materializes.

The ongoing process of desiring the outcome emerges from the individual's innate desiring process, and is less distinct and less ritualized than the highly specific ritual of bindling. Desiring the outcome is something that just kind of happens on its own on an ongoing basis, so long as the individual is allowing desire to flow within the self.

At the same time, because bindling provides the individual with the ability to desire the outcome with confidence, the individual who bindles can begin to desire the outcome in a more focused, deliberate way, with the understanding that doing so accelerates one's entry into the condition of inevitability.

The most effective way to focus one's innate, ongoing process of desiring the outcome while bindling, such that the desiring process optimally accelerates one's entry into the condition of inevitability, is through a process called paradoxical dual flooding.

180

Paradoxical Dual Flooding

Paradoxical dual flooding refers to paradoxical dual flooding of consciousness with (a) love of self exactly as is in the here and now and (b) visualized experiencing of the desired outcome.

In paradoxical dual flooding, the individual simultaneously floods consciousness fully with both of these components, with both complete love of self exactly as is in the here and now and with a visualized experience of the desired outcome.

This dual flooding process is paradoxical in that the individual loves and accepts the self entirely, such that the love and the self-acceptance are completely non-contingent on the desired outcome, yet at the same time the individual acknowledges and honors the presence in the psyche of desire for a specific bodily form, and channelizes this desire into the imaginative faculty of visualization.

Paradoxical dual flooding is the most effective way to accelerate one's entry into the condition of inevitability, the condition in which the desired outcome becomes inevitable and materializes, because it directly strengthens the powerful charge between the individual and the desired outcome.

Note that the two components of the paradoxical dual flooding process are directly connected with the two components of the powerful charge, i.e., with the individual and with the desired outcome. Specifically, love of self exactly as is in the here and now is directly connected with the individual, and visualized experiencing of the desired outcome is directly connected with the desired outcome.

Paradoxical dual flooding is a powerful process because it links together the individual and the desired outcome, strengthens the power of the charge between them, and thereby magnetizes them together and merges them such that the individual and the desired outcome become one.

Desire is a raw manifestation of the creative process within the self, and as such, it is very powerful. Paradoxical dual flooding channelizes the innate power of desire into the process of materializing the desired outcome. Paradoxical dual flooding is desire effectively channelized, because it is a desiring process in which the desire serves to strengthen the charge between the individual and the desired outcome.

Ineffectively channelized desire, on the other hand, is any desiring process that does not strengthen a charge between the individual and a desired outcome, and therefore does not actually bring a desired outcome closer to materializing.

Ineffectively channelizing one's desiring process is a waste of life energy, and because desire is powerful, focusing one's desiring process in a way that does not actually contribute to the materialization of a desired outcome can actually result in making the individual quite miserable.

When the individual bindles and simultaneously desires the outcome through paradoxical dual flooding, the individual's innate desiring process is effectively channelized, such that it serves to strengthen the charge between the individual and the desired outcome and thus to bring the individual into the condition of inevitability.

Paradoxical dual flooding involves simultaneous flooding of consciousness with (a) love of self exactly as is in the here and now and (b) visualized experiencing of the desired outcome.

Love of self exactly as is in the here and now

Love of self exactly as is in the here and now is the first and foundational component of paradoxical dual flooding.

Love of self exactly as is in the here and now is the innate, original condition and process of the psyche. When allowed to function unfettered, love of self exactly as is in the here and now circulates on its own throughout the entirety of the psyche.

Love of self exactly as is in the here and now is a manifestation of the creative process within the individual, and as such, it is a very powerful process. The full power of the divine, the full power of the creative process, is manifested in the process of love of self exactly as is in the here and now.

In allowing the process of love of self exactly as is in the here and now to flow freely within the psyche, the individual is allowing the creative process itself to flow freely within the psyche. As this creative energy is allowed to circulate freely within the psyche, the psyche remains open and receptive to the development of the powerful charge between the individual and the desired outcome, wherein the individual and the desired outcome become one.

Although love of self exactly as is in the here and now is the innate, original condition and process of the psyche, it is possible for the love of self process to become compromised by the individual superimposing shame and should upon the psyche.

When love of self exactly as is in the here and now becomes compromised through the imposition of shame and should on the psyche, the movements of the creative process within the psyche become blocked, and the love of self process gets locked up inside a very small prison cell somewhere inside the psyche. The imprisoned love of self process thus becomes prevented from circulating throughout the psyche in its fullness, and the psyche as a whole enters into a condition of stuckness and inertia, a condition that is highly conducive to the retention of excess weight.

While it is possible to restrict the range of motion of the love of self process by confining it to this lone, solitary prison cell, it is impossible to bring this innate process into complete inertia and to prevent it from moving entirely. Movement is the most basic, universal quality of the creative process, and the innate love of self process is a manifestation of the creative process. Therefore, while love of self can be confined and restricted, it can never be fully banished from the psyche.

Love of self exactly as is in the here and now is the heroic drive within the psyche, and even when imprisoned, it will continue to move around within the prison cell to which it has been confined, and will continually do everything it possibly can to break

184

free and return to its full range of motion, i.e., to return to circulating freely throughout the psyche in its entirety.

As long as the individual continues to cling to shame and should that have been superimposed on the psyche, love of self exactly as is in the here and now will remain imprisoned within this prison cell inside the psyche.

Over time the individual may have become so habituated to shame and should as to have gotten to a point of believing that the superimposed shame and should are innate to the psyche, and that the innate love of self exactly as is in the here and now is superimposed. If this is the case, and if the individual is surrounded by others in a culture that has become habituated to shame and should, then even the very idea of love of self may seem corny, false, and contrived.

Once we come to the self-evident realization that love of self exactly as is in the here and now is the innate, original condition and process of the psyche, and that it is shame and should that are superimposed on the psyche—and that the superimposed shame and should are responsible for imprisoning the love of self process—it then becomes easy for us to release shame and should, and to fully facilitate and embrace love of self exactly as is in the here and now.

When we release shame and should and fully facilitate and embrace love of self exactly as is in the here and now, we release love of self from the prison cell into which it has been restricted, and from which it has been attempting to break free on our behalf.

After love of self is released from the prison cell, it begins to move around and to explore and rediscover the psyche. It moves around here and there and everywhere, throughout the heights, the depths, and the many various interconnecting channels of the psyche. It flows out and finds its way back into all of these neglected areas, and begins to circulate throughout all of these areas.

As the love of self process gets back into its full circulation, the task of the individual is simply to allow this process to occur, to facilitate this process and to stay out of its way. The individual does this simply by dwelling entirely in ecstasy and desire, and by protecting and honoring these innate processes of ecstasy and desire as they operate in union with the innate, original process of love of self exactly as is in the here and now.

As love of self exactly as is in the here and now begins to move around throughout the entirety of the psyche, the individual begins to move out of inertia, such that the life of the individual comes to be characterized by continual, gentle, ongoing movement. The psyche becomes highly receptive to the development of the powerful charge between the individual and the desired outcome, wherein the desired outcome becomes inevitable and materializes.

As love of self exactly as is in the here and now begins to move around throughout the psyche, in all areas of the psyche, the individual enters into the depths of mystic experience.

It is within the inner depths of the psyche of the individual that the individual encounters the divine directly. This is where the

186

individual comes into direct communion with the creative process, of which the individual is a divine manifestation.

The individual becomes enraptured in a deep, loving relationship with the creative process, a deep, loving relationship with the self as a divine manifestation of the creative process.

The chemistry in this relationship is deep, intense, powerful, and very fulfilling.

The ongoing love of self process is an ongoing, automatic process in the sense that the individual simply facilitates this process and allows it to occur. At the same time, the individual is a romanced, enchanted partner in this loving relationship, and is able to do all kinds of sweet, loving things to the self, such as whispering sweet nothings to the self, gently caressing one's own body, and so on.

When love of self exactly as is in the here and now becomes fully manifested in the psyche and in the life of the individual, it then becomes possible for the individual to become enthroned as the protagonist in the individual's own life.

Love of self exactly as is in the here and now: Loving the body

When the individual wishes to effortlessly release excess weight and permanently maintain desired bodily form, it becomes particularly necessary for the individual's love of self exactly as is in the here and now to include love of the individual's body exactly as it is in the here and now.

Loving one's own body exactly as it is in the here and now is something the individual may vehemently resist, especially if the individual has become deeply accustomed to viewing the body through a lens of shame.

The thing is, effortless releasing of excess weight and permanent maintenance of desired bodily form literally is not possible until the individual finds a way to love the body exactly as it is in the here and now.

The easiest way to begin loving the body exactly as it is in the here and now is to begin viewing it with the same neutrality with which one views any of the forms and elements that make up the universe.

The human body is a manifestation of the divine that is, simultaneously, a mere accretion of elements. To view the body in this way is to recognize that it is continuous with all of the elements in the universe, in all of their manifested forms and conditions.

The self-portrait (optional). One possible way of deepening one's connection with this realization—the realization that the human body is a manifestation of the divine that is continuous with all of the elements in the universe—is to create a self-portrait.

The creation of a self-portrait facilitates a deliberate, systematic bypassing of the judging part of the brain that has retained learned ideas of shame and should in regard to the body.

The creation of a self-portrait allows the individual to instead practice using the sensorial faculties, to become immersed in direct sensorial experience, and to thereby directly view the divine essence embodied in one's material form.

In creating a self-portrait, the individual replicates divine essence and simultaneously experiences a mystic connection with this essence. This experience deepens the individual's connection with the transpersonal and the universal, and provides the individual with a means of directly witnessing one's true identity as an actual manifestation of the divine, an actual manifestation of the creative process. In creating a self-portrait, the individual is able to fully metabolize this understanding of one's innately divine nature.

Deliberately ignoring the judging part of one's brain is essential for the individual to encounter the divine while creating a self-portrait. Approaching a self-portrait in this way involves drawing in the same way children draw, by simply relaxing and enjoying the process and creating a genuine replication of what is seen.

Deliberately bypassing the judging part of the brain in this way makes it easier for the individual to release learned ideas of shame and should, and to become more deeply connected with one's inherent divinity and continuity with all of the elements, forms, and processes that constitute the universe.

Sensorial people watching. If at first the individual encounters some difficulty in loving one's own body exactly as it is in the here and now, a good way to begin to facilitate the releasing of shame is to participate in some sensorial people watching.

Sensorial people watching is a simple practice, and is something to have fun with. It involves deliberately finding a way of detaching from the weary pattern of looking at people and their bodies through an evaluative lens, and instead viewing them in an entirely sensorial manner.

While looking at bodies in a sensorial manner, the individual deliberately refrains from categorizing various human forms as good or bad, beautiful or ugly, and so on, and simply becomes absorbed in the basic, non-judging sensorial perception of the image of a person, in all its details and qualities, as this image is processed in the visual system of the viewer.

Judgments about bodies are learned, so these need only be released. The experience of fully sensorily processing the image of a person without applying any judgments to the experience is primal and powerful mystic experience. It brings the individual into direct contact with the divine, underlying presence that interconnects and unites all that is.

As the individual begins to experience this direct connection with the divine, it then becomes easier for the individual to recognize the self as a manifestation of the divine, and to fully facilitate and embrace the innate, original process of love of self exactly as is in the here and now.

Visualized experiencing of the desired outcome

The second component of the paradoxical dual flooding process is visualized experiencing of the desired outcome.

Visualized experiencing of the desired outcome is a highly individualized process wherein the individual finds a way to playfully tap into the inner imaginative process of visualization in such a way that the individual is able to experience in the mind the full sensorial experience of the desired outcome being delivered to the self and becoming fully manifested in the life of the individual.

Visualized experiencing of the desired outcome is a highly effective process because the psyche is malleable, receptive, and magical. The psyche is the creator of dreams that completely defy what the individual considers to be possible in waking life.

In visualized experiencing of the desired outcome, the individual taps directly into the place of dreaming. The place of dreaming is the place in the mind where dreams are made. It is the imagination, the realm of fantasy. It is the mind of the child, the part of the self that believes anything is possible. This part of the self is powerful and is just as real as any other aspect of reality.

When the individual experiences the desired outcome in fantasy, through visualized experiencing of the desired outcome, the individual experiences the desired outcome in this very real place, in the place of dreaming within the psyche. To the psyche, an experience that occurs in the place of dreaming is just as real as an experience that occurs in everyday waking life.

Therefore, as the individual bathes in the fantasy of the desired outcome on a regular basis within the place of dreaming, while simultaneously loving the self exactly as is in the here and now, the powerful charge between the individual and the desired outcome seeps into the psyche at its deepest levels, saturates the psyche through and through, and dissolves any and all resistance between the individual and the desired outcome.

Power Objects

Paradoxical dual flooding is particularly effective when it is facilitated through the use of power objects.

In the context of bindling, a power object is any object the individual creates or acquires that facilitates in the mind of the individual the simultaneous occurrence of both of the components of paradoxical dual flooding, (a) love of self exactly as is in the here and now and (b) visualized experiencing of the desired outcome.

The use of power objects is a deliberate, proactive approach to the desiring process wherein the individual creates and/or acquires specific objects that facilitate paradoxical dual flooding in the mind of the individual while the individual sensorily experiences these objects—for example, while holding (or holding onto), viewing, and contemplating any such object.

Use of power objects is a way of strengthening the powerful charge between the individual and the desired outcome and thereby accelerating one's entry into the condition of inevitability.

Examples

Collage. One example of a power object is a collage of images cut and pasted together by the individual, images that the individual has selected and combined because the viewing of these images facilitates simultaneous occurrence in the mind of the individual of both love of self exactly as is in the here and now and visualized experiencing of the desired outcome.

Vignette. Another example of a power object is a sheet of paper on which the individual has written out an imagined scenario in which the individual is experiencing the desired bodily form — a scenario that has been written in such a way that when the individual reads it, the individual fully experiences love of self exactly as is in the here and now and simultaneously experiences in visualization the desired outcome.

In both of these examples of power objects, imagery is a key component. Power objects that are used for paradoxical dual flooding are likely to include some type of imagery, given that imagery facilitates visualized experiencing of the desired outcome. As demonstrated in the examples above, imagery can be evoked in the mind both through the use of actual images and through the use of imagery-evoking text.

However, a power object does not necessarily need to include any type of image or imagery-evoking text in order to facilitate paradoxical dual flooding. A power object can be literally anything, provided it facilitates in the mind of the individual the full simultaneous occurrence of both components of paradoxical dual flooding. For example, an audio recording that facilitates paradoxical dual flooding in the mind of the individual can be used as a power object.

While I contemplate this object

The process of creating or acquiring a power object is a highly personal, individualized process, because the images and emotions that are evoked in the mind of one person by a specific power object may be completely different from the images and emotions that would be evoked in the mind of another person by that same object.

The key, central question to ask oneself throughout the process of creating and/or acquiring power objects is,

While I contemplate this object, am I fully experiencing love of self exactly as is in the here and now and simultaneously experiencing in visualization my desired outcome?

194

It is through asking oneself this question on an ongoing basis that the individual begins to discover what is and what is not a power object for oneself.

Therefore, in the process of creating or acquiring a power object, the key variable of interest is not the actual content of the object itself. Rather, the key variable of interest is what is happening in the mind of the individual while the individual is contemplating the object.

My first power object

The process of creating or acquiring one's first power object is something that begins as soon as one is introduced to the concept of a power object. It is a process that begins in the mind, as the individual begins to notice the degree to which various types of stimuli either do or do not facilitate in one's own mind the simultaneous occurrence of love of self exactly as is in the here and now and visualized experiencing of the desired outcome.

The creation or acquisition of one's first power object is something that is likely to just kind of happen on its own, as a function of the individual beginning to notice what does and what does not facilitate paradoxical dual flooding in one's own mind.

A collection of power objects

Once the individual has created or acquired one power object, a collection of multiple power objects may then naturally begin to form as the individual begins to notice other items in the environment and considers these items for possible acquisition or adaptation as power objects. The individual can then begin to have fun with the process of deciding on which items to acquire or adapt into one's collection of power objects.

Bringing together multiple power objects into a collection of power objects is a way of signifying that the objects are sacred and important to the self, and increases their overall potential to facilitate paradoxical dual flooding. This is true even in the case of power objects that are digital files on an electronic device: Bringing them together in a single location (e.g., within a single folder on one's computer) signifies their sacredness and importance to the self, and increases their overall power in relation to the psyche.

The formation of a collection of power objects is a playful process that can be thought of as the creating of a toy chest for the mind of the child that lives within the psyche of the adult. To fully facilitate one's entry into this playful process, the individual may wish to have some fun with the process of deciding on a suitable container for one's personal collection of power objects.

A container for a collection of power objects can be a box, a scrapbook, a blank book, or a folder on a computer. It can be something that is acquired or something that is created, or it can be something that is both acquired and created, such as a box that is acquired and then decorated to personalize it.

A container for a collection of power objects can be created or acquired either before the creation or acquisition of one's first power object or after one or more power objects have been collected.

A collection of power objects is something that is likely to change and evolve over time. For example, at some point the individual may find that an object that was once effective in facilitating paradoxical dual flooding is no longer effective in facilitating paradoxical dual flooding. In this case, the individual may wish to either remove the object from the collection or to find some way of altering the object so that it again fully facilitates paradoxical dual flooding.

Also, from time to time the individual may wish to alter the container in which a collection of power objects is kept, or to move one's collection of objects into a new container.

A process piece (optional)

One especially powerful way to approach the creation of a power object is to create a process-focused power object that facilitates paradoxical dual flooding and that simultaneously represents the individual's journey through the bindling process.

The most basic way of creating a process-focused power object is to create a sequenced series of 100 process-focused panels during 100 days of bindling. Examples of ways to create a sequence of 100 process-focused panels are as follows:

On each of 100 consecutive pages, the individual sketches a daily image that in some way facilitates paradoxical dual flooding and that simultaneously represents what is going on within the psyche of the individual on that day. This could be something along the lines of a mandala, or even just a simple daily drawing that is completed in a few seconds per day. It could also incorporate words and/or pasted-in images.

On each of 100 consecutive pages, the individual sketches a daily self-portrait that in some way facilitates paradoxical dual flooding within the mind of the individual. This could be a quick, rough sketch, or one that is more detailed. (Note that any created image can be thought of as a self-portrait; for example, a mandala can be thought of as a portrait of the psyche.)

On each of 100 consecutive days, the individual creates a daily, consecutively numbered self-photo that in some way facilitates paradoxical dual flooding within the mind of the individual. One benefit of creating a daily (or even a weekly or monthly), consecutively numbered self-photo is that it keeps the individual on the edge of the individual's seat, witnessing the desired bodily form as it actually materializes.

Unboxing Press publishes a book titled *Power Object*, which includes 100 blank pages and can therefore be used to create a series of 100 process-focused panels.

Blank book (optional)

A book such as *Power Object* that includes blank pages can be used by the individual who is bindling for the purpose of delving more deeply into the bindling process in all kinds of different ways, even apart from using it to create a sequenced series of 100 panels. For example, it can be used

to sketch out daily food selection ideas,

to record dreams,

for free-form exploration of images and ideas, reflections, insights, doodles, and so on,

to record recipes,

to plot out upcoming food indulgences,

to journal or write out ideas for new hobbies, projects, adventures, creative ideas, etc.,

to create lists—for example, a list of things the individual loves to do—things the individual will be able to do more of now that time and energy have been freed up in the life of the individual due to bindling,

and to document the changes that are beginning to occur in one's psyche and in one's life as a function of the deeper, underlying transformation of self process that is activated by the ritual of bindling.

A book such as *Power Object* can also just be left blank and enjoyed as is.

The Magic Door

Through the process of creating and/or acquiring one or more power objects, the individual begins to develop an awareness and an attunement to the specific types of stimuli that facilitate paradoxical dual flooding—and the specific types of stimuli that do not facilitate paradoxical dual flooding—within one's own psyche.

As a natural consequence of this evolving sensitivity to the ways in which various physical objects influence one's thoughts and one's emotions, the individual is likely to begin to become more aware of the degree to which various aspects of the personal spaces occupied by the individual—including spaces at home, at work, in the car, etc.—either do or do not facilitate paradoxical dual flooding.

As this awareness begins to increase within the individual, the individual may wish to begin to make some changes within these personal spaces so as to more fully facilitate paradoxical dual flooding. For example, the individual may wish to remove items that do not facilitate paradoxical dual flooding, to give greater prominence to items that do facilitate paradoxical dual flooding, and/or to make any other kind of change to facilitate the ongoing paradoxical dual flooding process. Items may be rearranged, new items may be brought into a space, walls may be repainted, and so on.

Any such changes that are made are made based on the individual's evolving awareness of how to facilitate paradoxical dual flooding in one's own mind—an awareness that begins to develop as a function of one's contemplation of one's first power object.

As soon as the individual makes one or two such changes in the individual's personal spaces, this signifies that the personal spaces of the individual are becoming a magic door. A magic door is a physical environment that is fully conducive to the process of paradoxical dual flooding within the psyche of the individual, and which thus fully facilitates one's entry into the condition of inevitability.

The formation of a magic door is the most important and the most significant progress point in the paradoxical dual flooding process, as it is in the formation of a magic door that the individual literally becomes flooded and fully engulfed in the paradoxical dual flooding process. In the formation of a magic door, the powerful charge between the individual and the desired outcome becomes fully embedded within the entirety of one's physical environment.

Focus on what goes on inside

The key to allowing one's personal spaces to become a magic door is to focus less on how one's personal spaces look or appear and to focus more on what goes on inside of oneself while one is in these spaces. This involves considering one's mental associations to items in one's spaces, the types of emotions and images aroused by various aspects of these spaces, memories that are evoked while in these spaces, and so on.

The actual appearances of one's spaces and of the items contained therein are important in that they influence the emotions and mental images that one experiences while in these spaces, but it is what actually goes on in one's emotions and in one's mind while one is in these spaces that is the variable of interest.

Await its formation

As the individual begins to observe the degree to which various aspects of one's personal spaces either do or do not facilitate paradoxical dual flooding, at some point an idea is likely to show up in the individual's mind regarding a specific change the individual could make in the physical environment that would more effectively facilitate the ongoing paradoxical dual flooding process.

Once such an idea shows up in the mind of the individual, the individual is under no obligation to immediately (or ever) act on this idea. Personal spaces and the items that are kept within these spaces are extensions of one's psyche, and as such they do not respond well to the individual rushing or pressuring the self to make changes within them. In fact, rushing or pressuring oneself to begin to form a magic door is likely to just stir up internal resistance to the natural unfolding of the process.

The most effective way to allow a magic door to form in one's personal spaces is to await the arrival in one's mind of a truly enticing or compelling idea regarding a possible change to make within one's personal spaces. A truly compelling idea possesses the ability to draw the individual into action, without any self-pressuring on the part of the individual.

The first idea that comes into the individual's mind about a possible change to make in one's personal spaces may not possess this enticing quality, and so the individual may need to wait for a truly enticing idea to show up, an idea that is so enticing and compelling that the idea itself draws the individual into action.

By focusing one's energy and attention only on ideas that are truly enticing, the individual dwells entirely in ecstasy and desire throughout the formation of the magic door process. When the individual dwells entirely in ecstasy and desire in this way, the individual works in the deepest possible cooperation with the psyche, such that all resistance dissolves, and the magic door forms on its own.

Also, when the individual dwells entirely in ecstasy and desire throughout the formation of the magic door process, the full ongoing circulation of the innate processes of ecstasy and desire becomes seamlessly embedded into the magic door itself, and thus into the psyche and the life of the individual.

Once one truly enticing idea shows up in the individual's mind regarding a possible change to make in one's personal spaces—an idea that is so compelling that the idea itself draws the individual into action—more enticing ideas begin to show up in the mind of the individual, and the individual likewise becomes drawn into taking action on these ideas as well. The magic door then almost automatically begins to materialize in full surround of the individual.

Releasing disempowering objects

In the formation of a magic door within one's personal spaces, it may require some courage to get rid of disempowering objects, i.e., to get rid of anything that in any way does not facilitate paradoxical dual flooding.

The individual reserves the right to only retain objects that make the individual feel good to the core—items that the individual truly loves, and that fully facilitate the ongoing paradoxical dual flooding process.

The individual is under no obligation to possess anything, really, except maybe a few vital documents and an article of clothing to prevent getting arrested for public nudity.

It is very liberating to only retain objects that make the individual feel good to the core, items that are beloved, treasured, special, and powerful—items that fully facilitate paradoxical dual flooding.

The bindling ritual establishes a precedent for thinking of one's possessions in this way, given that in the bindling ritual the individual specifies and eats only treasured, deeply enjoyed items.

The individual may discover that one's body and one's belongings tend to operate in a parallel process; specifically, as the individual becomes more willing to let go of disempowering, unwanted objects that occupy the individual's personal spaces, in a parallel process the body of the individual may become more willing to release the excess weight it had been retaining.

The individual is under no obligation to retain objects for historical purposes. Examination of any culture reveals that history is an ongoing revisionary process, that history itself is a process of revising and reframing the story of a group of people. Therefore, editing one's possessions is a way of taking up authorship of one's own life, of claiming ownership of self, and of weaving together a revised life narrative that is conducive with the innermost desires of the individual.

The recreated space

Over time the individual may discover that it is often much easier to acquire possessions than it is to release them and let them go. Therefore, as the individual becomes engaged in the process of creating a magic door in all spaces occupied by the individual, all of these spaces become sacred, and the individual becomes more selective about the specific items that the individual chooses to allow into these spaces.

As the magic door process develops, the individual may wish to receive a consultation regarding one's personal spaces from a person who has demonstrated success in helping individuals to bring their personal spaces into alignment with their desired outcomes. A good consultant provides the individual with a perceptive bird's eye assessment of the individual's life and personal spaces, a view that the individual may not otherwise perceive due to being embedded within one's own life situation.

Power Objects and a Magic Door – As Innately Desired

The use of power objects and the formation of a magic door are really only effective when the individual participates in these processes when the individual innately desires to do so.

The purpose of these processes is to facilitate the innate circulation of desire within the individual; use of power objects and the formation of a magic door are ways of channelizing desire when desire is experienced, such that the charge between the individual and the desired outcome gains strength.

Therefore, participation in these processes is never an extra "to do" task. It is simply an option, a pleasurable way of channelizing desire that is available to the individual for whenever desire arises from within the self.

Use of power objects and the formation of a magic door are processes that accelerate the individual's entry into the condition of inevitability, but it is only bindling that is the core, foundational, daily process.

When desire for the outcome does arise from within the self, there is never any obligation to channelize it into use of power objects or into the formation of a magic door. Sometimes it feels good to feel desire and to just feel it, to simply soak it in and bask in it.

The key to success in the use of power objects and in the formation of a magic door is to maintain a stance of paradoxical detached attachment with these processes—to have fun engaging with these processes when there is an innate desire to do so, but otherwise to forget about them and get on with other things.

Use of power objects and the formation of a magic door are powerful processes, and the effects of any participation in either of these processes will continue to churn on their own on an ongoing basis deep within the psyche, while the individual is getting on with other stuff.

Everyone and Everything

Through the ongoing use of power objects and the formation of a magic door, the individual comes to experience paradoxical dual flooding on a continual, ongoing basis, including during times when the individual is not deliberately focused on doing so. Paradoxical dual flooding comes to be a continual, ongoing process that the individual merely witnesses occurring within one's psyche and in one's life.

Through this ongoing paradoxical dual flooding process, all aspects of the life of the individual come to be aligned in accordance with the desired outcome being delivered to the self. One important manifestation of this comprehensive alignment that develops between the individual and the desired outcome is that the individual acquires a newfound ability to receive inspiration from everyone and everything.

Therefore, if at any time the individual ends up in a situation that feels uninspiring, the individual is able to view this as a fun challenge presenting itself to the individual, a challenge to find a way of deriving inspiration and benefit from the situation. The individual thereby becomes able to experience communion with the creative process in any situation the individual encounters.

It can be especially challenging to find a way to derive inspiration from a situation in which a ritual is occurring wherein the person or persons facilitating the ritual are deliberately trying to arouse feelings of inspiration in those who are present in a way that feels corny or contrived, or when the desired outcomes of the facilitators are not in alignment with the desired outcomes of the individual.

In situations of this nature, the individual is able to transcend the situation and experience communion with the creative process by doing some simple mental cutting and pasting. This involves simply editing out in one's mind the parts that are not conducive with the values of the individual, and (mentally) filling in the individual's desired outcome and ideas that are conducive with the values of the individual.

In this way, the individual is able to reject the agenda of the facilitators while still absorbing the energy of inspiration and channelizing this energy into the individual's own process of receiving a desired outcome from the creative process.

Desired Outcome

When the individual participates in the ritual of bindling, the individual turns over the task of effortlessly releasing excess weight and permanently maintaining desired bodily form to the creative process as it is manifested in the deeper levels of the psyche.

Then, one day the individual wakes up and discovers that the body has been transformed.

In the process of effortlessly releasing excess weight, the individual experiences the desired transformation in a series of stages that the individual is able to demarcate according to the specific days on which the individual wakes up and discovers specific physical evidence of the creative process having done its work in bringing the desired outcome one step closer to its full materialization.

The periodic occurrence of such days is deeply rewarding to the individual, and reinforces and energizes the ongoing daily bindling process.

This ongoing process continues along, and then one day the individual wakes up and discovers that the desired outcome, the individual's desired bodily form, has been delivered.

Integration

When the desired outcome is delivered to the individual, the individual may feel more exposed and vulnerable without the additional layers of padding and protection that formerly surrounded the body. It is important therefore for the individual to keep the transformed body warm, cushioned, and protected on an ongoing basis.

For example, in cooler climates, seasons, and buildings (e.g., due to air conditioning), the individual may need to begin wearing additional layers of clothing to keep the body warm. Also, sitting one's weight-released body on a hard chair is likely to be a much more pleasant experience when the individual first places a cushion on the chair.

Keeping the body comfortable on an ongoing basis by carefully attending to bodily temperature and cushioning is an expression of love of self exactly as is in the here and now.

214

Attending to one's ongoing comfort level in this way eliminates any reasons for the body to acquire excess weight and communicates to the psyche at its deepest levels that the individual views the desired bodily form as permanent and wishes for the body to remain in this condition.

Also, fully welcoming the desired outcome into one's life involves fully embracing ecstasy as a way of life. This involves continually treating oneself to a wide range of pleasurable experiences that are not necessarily food-related. For example, from time to time the individual may wish to indulge in a hot bath, or in a massage, or in a simple walk out into the woods, and so on.

The Miracle of Movement

When the individual starts out in the bindling process, there is no need to simultaneously come up with an exercise plan to accompany the dieting process. The miracle of bindling is that it places the individual into a condition in which movement or exercising of the body begins to ripple out on its own, effortlessly, as an innately desired manifestation of the creative process.

This ripple effect occurs as an automatic function of the individual entering into the sacred space of self-mastery and staying out of the way while the creative process carries out a deep and complete transformation of the psyche and the life of the individual.

The transformation of self process itself is characterized by the initiation of deep levels of movement deep within the psyche, deep automatic movements that then ripple out in a literal, physical way, throughout the body of the individual.

The transformation of self process gains increasing momentum as energy that was formerly trapped in the unrewarding cycles of willy nilly eating is released, and as energy that was formerly stuck in the inertia of shame and should is released.

All of this released energy gets channelized into the transformation of self process and ripples out into actual physical movements in the body of the individual.

The transformation of self process also lays down a template wherein the psyche becomes optimally configured to facilitate the perpetual ongoing movements of the creative process—of which the individual is a literal manifestation—throughout the body and the life of the individual.

Movement is the most basic, universal quality of the creative process. It is the universal miracle. We have yet to discover a single location in the universe where anything remains stationary. This is as true for entire galaxies as it is for subatomic particles.

When the individual bindles, the individual simply creates an optimal situation wherein this innate, universal movement of the creative process is facilitated in rippling throughout the body of the individual. In this process there is no need whatsoever for the individual to engage in any pushing or pulling of the self. The individual simply becomes positioned or aligned in such a way that the innate movements of the creative process flow throughout the body of the individual on a continual, ongoing basis.

One way to conceptualize effortless movement is to think about the feeling of standing up after having been cramped into a small seat on an airplane for several hours. After having had one's body stuck in such a small, cramped space for so long, when the individual finally stands up and stretches, it requires no effort at all. To the individual it actually feels as if the movement itself is pulling the individual into the motion, such that it is staying still that would require the exertion of effort.

There are endless possible ways in which the individual may channelize the movements of the creative process as these movements ripple throughout the body in an ecstatic, effortless manner. For example, the individual may feel an innate desire to take the stairs instead of the elevator, or to park in a less crowded area of the parking lot and enjoy a longer walk to the store.

What the individual gradually begins to discover is that moving around feels good, and that doing a little extra moving here and there is a way of gently increasing one's daily experience of pleasure. Doing a little extra moving here and there need not require any additional expenditure of time, and in many cases it actually saves time.

For example, parking farther away from the store saves time from a compulsive search for the closest possible parking spot, and sometimes taking the elevator actually requires more time than taking the stairs, especially when the elevator stops on multiple consecutive floors.

As the individual gradually begins to discover the pleasures of facilitating the movements of the creative process as these movements ripple throughout the body, the individual may wish to begin participating in more intensive forms of movement, given that more intensive forms of movement are highly conducive to facilitating the ecstatic psychospiritual condition of paradoxical mindful mindlessness.

For example, the individual may feel an innate desire to leap up stairs two at a time, to go on long, exciting, inspiring hikes, to play various sports, to lift weights, and so on.

More intensive forms of movement such as these possess the potential to bring the individual into extraordinarily deep, extended states of euphoria and ecstasy that go completely outside the bounds of ordinary human experience, states that ripple out and thrill and ripple out and thrill the brain and the entirety of the body, states that ripple out and thrill and ripple out and thrill the psyche of the individual at its very deepest levels, with extended, lingering effects, and no crash.

Movement is the most basic, universal quality of the creative process. It is the universal miracle. As the individual channelizes this basic quality of the creative process, the creative process then begins to open up endless potential pathways to adventure and ecstasy in the life of the individual.

The Creative Process

The individual is a manifestation of the creative process, a manifestation of the divine.

I am that I am.

Therefore, it is really only possible for the individual to be truly content while the individual is creating in one way or another.

When we are creating we are allowing the creative process to flow through us, and it is in this way that we create meaning. We create meaning by creating something, by channelizing the creative process as it flows through us into the composition of a specific form.

Participating in the flowing of the creative process in this way fulfills the deepest yearnings of the psyche and brings the individual into direct contact with the resplendence of the void, and with the joy and fun of being alive.

All that is is a series of creative processes.

All that is is a manifestation of the creative process.

When the individual becomes initiated into the process of bindling, the individual becomes initiated into a process of liberation, a process in which a specific type of limitation is introduced to the self as a means of freeing up energy within the psyche and in the life of the individual.

The individual who bindles becomes freed from having to think about what to eat except during the brief, few-minutes-daily bindling ritual. Time that was previously spent ruminating about what to eat, grazing around willy nilly, pacing back and forth to the fridge, and so on—all of that time becomes reduced to the brief, few-minutes-daily bindling ritual.

Also, on a deeper level, the individual who bindles becomes freed up from ever again having to worry or be concerned about the task of releasing excess weight and permanently maintaining desired bodily form. This task gets turned over to the creative process, and the desired outcome becomes automatically programmed into the life of the individual.

The time and energy that are freed up in the life of the individual who bindles then become available to the individual, to be channelized into whatever sorts of dreams, pursuits, hobbies, passions, and so on, that the individual may have been harboring for all these years.

This freeing up of creative energy that occurs as a function of the bindling process provides the individual with the opportunity of a lifetime in the sense that it opens up the life of the individual to all kinds of new possibilities and adventures. At the same time, taking full advantage of this opportunity of a lifetime is highly adaptive in that it provides a channel into which the energy that is freed up by the bindling process can effortlessly flow.

If the individual releases creative energy by bindling and then just lets this energy sit there in a state of entropy, the released energy will absolutely refuse to sit still, and may begin to express itself in the form of cravings for excess food.

This energy that becomes freed up as a function of bindling is a raw manifestation of the creative process, and as such, its most basic quality is movement. It will always move, and if we do not provide it with a channel into which it is able to flow, then it will find some other way to express itself.

This is why it is almost never a good idea to just kind of sit around and think in an aimless sort of way, in a state of entropy. It is almost always better for the psyche to have some type of deliberate activity or ritual into which energy and attention can be focused, to remain engaged with some kind of activity or ritual on a continual, ongoing basis. This can be something as simple as a breathing meditation, or knitting, or building a train set, or playing a video game.

Keeping oneself gently engaged with some type of deliberate activity or ritual on an ongoing basis does not require any sort of pushing or pulling of the self. It is simply a matter of providing for oneself a channel into which one's continually flowing life energy is able to flow.

The simplest way to provide oneself with this channel is to continually provide oneself, from moment to moment, with a series of low to moderate energy level activities.

Low to moderate energy level activities occupy a cozy liminal space, a cozy sweet spot, between inertia and higher intensity movement. Getting oneself into this cozy sweet spot of low to moderate energy level activity provides the psyche with a baseline foundation, a basic foundational way of spending and enjoying the majority of one's time.

221

Then, once the individual gets out of inertia and into this cozy sweet spot, at times the individual may wish to take it up a notch and participate in some higher intensity movement, as a means of increasing one's experience of ecstasy.

Low to moderate energy level activities provide for the psyche a space in which the creative energy that is released by the bindling process is able to move around and circulate on an ongoing basis. At the same time, keeping the psyche engaged in this way satisfies the most basic need of the psyche, i.e., its need to remain engaged with the creative process on a continual, ongoing basis.

As the individual becomes immersed in low to moderate energy level activities on a continual, ongoing basis, the individual experiences a gentle engagement with whatever the task at hand may be. The individual enters into the deepest levels of relaxation and experiences subtle stimulation and pleasure on a continual, ongoing basis.

Some low to moderate energy level activities result in the creation of a finished product, and some do not. Some are simply a pleasant way of passing the time, such as playing a game of cards or going for a walk. It isn't necessary to always be doing something that leads to a finished product. Life can be enjoyed just as is. We aren't machines. What is necessary, simply, is to experience continual, ongoing engagement with the creative process.

Television viewing is an activity that can be highly pleasurable provided the individual feels engaged with the activity in some way, for example, through some form of ritualization. Another option is to take it up a notch by playing a video game, an activity that can be used to stimulate the psyche's innate striving for movement and adventure, so that movement and adventure can then begin to gradually spread into various aspects of one's life.

When the individual becomes initiated into the process of bindling, the energy that was formerly wrapped up in willy nilly eating becomes freed up, and the individual is able then to redirect this energy into low to moderate energy level activities that provide ongoing pleasure to the individual and that occupy that cozy liminal sweet spot between inertia and high intensity movement.

A lot of the willy nilly eating of excess food that may have occurred prior to the individual's initiation into the bindling process may have been due simply to the individual being bored and not feeling engaged and absorbed in an activity of interest.

Boredom then is not so much boredom per se, rather it is the innate, ongoing need for the psyche to be occupied, to be engaged in pleasant, absorbing activities on a continual, ongoing basis — even if this is something as simple as a breathing meditation.

If, prior to bindling, this need for continual, ongoing engagement was not being met, then the psyche may have created its own form of engagement through the willy nilly eating of excess food.

Once the individual becomes initiated into the process of bindling, the energy that was previously wrapped up in willy nilly eating of excess food becomes freed up, and is in need of becoming engaged with pleasant, absorbing activities on a continual, ongoing basis.

While it is true that this newly available creative energy does in fact need to be redirected into engaging activities on a continual, ongoing basis, once we get this energy moving in this direction, we can then step back and really begin to take in the realization that in satisfying this need, we are at the same time experiencing the opportunity of a lifetime.

The creative energy that becomes freed up as a function of bindling is a raw manifestation of the creative process. This raw creative potential is a most precious commodity, a resource of the highest value that becomes available to the individual as a function of the bindling process.

This newly available resource can be thought of as money that needs to be spent. Creative energy is delivered to the individual as a function of bindling, and the individual then gets to have the pleasure of deciding exactly how to spend it.

The individual who bindles is particularly well positioned to figure out the best possible ways to use the creative energy that becomes freed up as a function of the bindling process. The individual who bindles experiences the deepest possible alteration of consciousness, one that results not only in the enhancement of ecstasy but also in the enhancement of insight and perception. Through the lens of this enhanced insight and perception, the individual begins to discover ways of channelizing this newly available creative energy such that this energy deepens ecstasy in the life of the individual and leads to the effortless materialization of desired outcomes.

The process of figuring out one's own personal creative path is an experience of deep communion with the creative process. It is something that the individual both directs and witnesses. In this process of deep communion, the will of the individual directs the ways in which the creative process is channelized, and at the same time, the universal power of the creative process enters into and transforms the life and even the will of the individual. The individual and the universal become one, and the individual experiences an atonement with the individual's true nature as an innately divine manifestation of the creative process.

The freeing up of creative energy that the individual experiences as a function of the bindling process provides the individual with an opportunity to try out that one thing the individual has always dreamed of trying. Then, if the individual tries out "that one thing" and it doesn't pan out for whatever reason, the discovery of this outcome is a success in and of itself. The individual is then able to say, "I tried that, it didn't pan out, so now let's move on to the next idea."

The individual can make a list of things to try, keep adding to the list as new ideas appear in the mind, and then just keep moving down the list until something clicks. This in itself is an adventure and a creative process.

The key to success in the process of discovering one's own personal creative path is to allow it to be an experimental, exploratory process, to take plenty of deep breaths and relax fully, and then just go with the flow and have fun with it.

The simple act of initiating the process of discovering one's creative path—for example, by starting a list of things to try—immediately brings the individual into direct, deep communion with the creative process. The fact that the path is not yet fully figured out is actually what makes it exciting. This is what makes it a true adventure. Half the fun is observing and witnessing as the creative process itself figures out, on the individual's behalf, a specific type of creative process that is conducive to the constitution of the individual.

Bindling does in fact provide the individual with a monumental opportunity in that it frees up creative energy that the individual may then channelize into the discovery of a new creative path. The key though to taking full advantage of this monumental opportunity and figuring out one's own creative path is to approach this monumental opportunity in a very non-monumental way—i.e., to just start a list and start going through the list until something clicks.

A list of things to try can include pretty much anything. It might include items that are obviously creative, like learning a new musical instrument or doing cross-stitch, and also it might include items that are less obviously creative, like starting a new business or going back to school. It could be a project, a goal, a hobby, or an adventure. The possibilities are as endless as the manifestations of the creative process that span across the full expanse of the universe.

The key to success is to just keep moving down one's list until something clicks. An activity that clicks is an activity that easily facilitates in the individual the ecstatic psychospiritual condition of paradoxical mindful mindlessness.

In paradoxical mindful mindlessness, the individual is able to zone out and to simultaneously tune in to a deeper level of communion with the creative process. The individual enters into the condition of paradoxical mindful mindlessness by filling the mind entirely with the present moment activity and all of its nuances in their fullness. This complete filling of the mind and complete absorption in the present moment activity facilitates a paradoxical emptying and clearing out of the mind.

The psychospiritual condition of paradoxical mindful mindlessness is pleasant, soothing, fun, and enjoyable. When the individual enters into this condition on a deep level, hours could pass in what seem like minutes. Activities that are most conducive to paradoxical mindful mindlessness tend to be simple, repetitious, and fully absorbing of the attention and energy of the individual.

With experience the individual becomes able to experience paradoxical mindful mindlessness continually, at will, as this is the way in which the individual lives in continual communion with the creative process.

The initial entry point though for beginning to experience paradoxical mindful mindlessness is to discover a specific type of creative process that the individual enjoys, and which easily facilitates in the individual the psychospiritual condition of paradoxical mindful mindlessness.

This initial entry point then becomes a starting point wherein the individual is able to begin to experience ever-deepening levels of paradoxical mindful mindlessness, and to thereby experience deep communion with the creative process on a continual, ongoing basis.

When the mind enters into the condition of paradoxical mindful mindlessness, it becomes focused, serene, and enchanted. It is through this condition that the individual comes into direct encounter with the divine presence that animates all that is, and experiences directly the true nature of the self as an innately divine manifestation of this universal presence.

Magical as it is to experience paradoxical mindful mindlessness, it is helpful to keep in mind that it almost always take a little priming for an activity that is conducive to paradoxical mindful mindlessness to click.

Entering into paradoxical mindful mindlessness is similar to the process of priming a pump: The process begins with the initial challenge of bringing liquid into the pump, but then once it starts to flow, the process takes over and continues on its own.

All worthwhile creative processes that are truly, deeply rewarding to the individual require the discomfort of an initiation process, a process of priming the pump. To prime the pump in a creative process, the first step is for the individual to accept the fact that a potentially rewarding activity may feel boring and even unpleasant at first. Once this basic acceptance of the nature of a potentially rewarding activity has been established, the next step then is simply to get started, i.e., to just start going through the motions.

Then, at some point something magical happens. Something clicks. The pump becomes primed, and the process takes over and moves forward, seemingly of its own accord. The individual becomes caught up in a state of creative rapture and becomes as it were an observer of the creative process moving through the self.

Because the individual who bindles is facilitating in the psyche a gradually increasing condition of paradoxical mindful mindlessness, it becomes easy for the individual to approach the task of discovering a personal creative path with the highly adaptive stance of paradoxical detached attachment. With this stance, the individual is able to reflect on and engage with possibilities and ideas with a sense of playful detachment, wherein the individual engages with the ideas without ever taking them too seriously. This paradoxical stance actually allows the ideas to be crafted and re-crafted by the deeper magic of the creative process, and keeps the individual out of the way as this occurs.

Journaling — itself a creative act — is one of the best ways to figure out one's creative path, or at least to figure out the next step to take in figuring out one's creative path. It is a great way to explore in words one's innermost thoughts, desires, and yearnings, and to thereby discover items to add to one's list of things to try.

The creative path of the individual actually begins to open up in the very moment in which the individual begins to reflect on it. The individual simply steps into this process, and then witnesses as it unfolds and develops.

229

The individual is a manifestation of the creative process, a manifestation of the divine.

To bindle is to deliberately live in deep communion with the creative process. When the individual deliberately lives in deep communion with the creative process, the individual begins to discover ways in which the creative process is manifested in all aspects of life.

I am that I am.

So it is.

Three-Day Initiation Cycle

Now it is time for us to enter into the sacred space of self-mastery through the Three-Day Initiation Cycle.

The three days in the Three-Day Initiation Cycle are (1) the Pre-Liminal Day, (2) the Liminal Day, and (3) the Initiation Day. Note that in the ritual of bindling, days are divided by sleep cycles (not from midnight to midnight).

Each of these three days is represented by a separate one-page form on the pages that immediately follow this chapter. The three initiation forms are followed by a series of daily bindling forms, for 100 consecutive days of bindling.

Unboxing Press also publishes booklets of bindling forms that are available for purchase separately. These separately published booklets are available in two formats, the basic version and the advanced version.

Basic Forms. The basic version is identical to the set of bindling forms included at the end of this chapter. These basic forms include forms for the Three-Day Initiation Cycle and 100 days of bindling. Therefore, either the forms included in this book or a separate booklet of basic forms can be used for the Three-Day Initiation Cycle and 100 days of bindling. Booklets of basic forms can be identified by one black horizontal stripe that wraps around the upper portion of the booklet cover.

Advanced Forms. The advanced version is for individuals who have completed the Three-Day Initiation Cycle and remained within the sacred space of self-mastery for 100 days. The advanced forms are mostly identical to the basic forms; the one difference is that the advanced forms do not include forms for the initiation process. Initiated individuals may use the advanced forms for Days 101 to 200, Days 201 to 300, and so on. Booklets of advanced forms can be identified by two black horizontal stripes that wrap around the upper portion of the booklet cover.

The forms for each of the three days in the Three-Day Initiation Cycle are identified as follows:

Pre-Liminal Day. The form for the Pre-Liminal Day is indicated by the words *"PRE-LIMINAL* DAY" that appear at the top of the form.

Liminal Day. The form for the Liminal Day is indicated by the words *"LIMINAL* DAY" that appear at the top of the form.

Initiation Day. The form for the Initiation Day appears on the page immediately following the page on which the form for the Liminal Day appears. The form for the Initiation Day is indicated by the image of a laurel wreath that appears at the top of the form.

The Initiation Day form symbolizes entry into the sacred space of self-mastery. All subsequent forms are identical to the Initiation Day form, and thus symbolize ongoing continuation in the sacred space of self-mastery.

PRE-LIMINAL DAY

The first day in the Three-Day Initiation Cycle is the Pre-Liminal Day.

The tasks completed on the Pre-Liminal Day are as follows:

1. Write today's date in YYMMDD format in the lower right-hand corner of the Pre-Liminal Day form.

2. Write tomorrow's date in the lower right-hand corner of the Liminal Day form.

3. Select a series of food items to be eaten on the Liminal Day. These items will be listed on the Liminal Day form.

    In the food selection process, make sure that it will be ridiculously easy to follow through with the designated plan. The basic and only challenge of the Liminal Day is that of following through with the designated, intended plan and thereby entering into the sacred space of self-

238

mastery. This in itself is challenge enough, and it is important that the individual not add to this challenge in any way.

The key to success on the Liminal Day is to set the bar extremely low, to go extremely easy on oneself, and to thereby make it a guaranteed that the individual will follow through with the designated plan.

Going easy on oneself is particularly important during the Three-Day Initiation Cycle. Transitions are always stressful for the psyche, so the key to success is to be very gentle with oneself and to keep the process as effortless as is possible.

In coming up with a plan for the Liminal Day, it may be helpful to sketch out ideas on a separate piece of paper or in an electronic document.

Select food items based on the following three categories:

Unlimited

> The unlimited category is for food items that the individual wishes to be able to consume in unlimited amounts. These are items that the individual is confident will not impede the process of effortlessly releasing excess weight and permanently maintaining desired bodily form, regardless of amounts consumed.

239

The individual may wish to think of some unlimited items as treats. Unlimited items do not need to be obtained prior to the Liminal Day, as the individual is free to consume unlimited items in any amount (including "none") on the Liminal Day.

Obtained

The obtained category is the main category in the bindling ritual, and allows for the highest level of specificity. Items that are listed in the obtained category on the Liminal Day form are obtained on the Pre-Liminal Day; in other words, they are obtained one day in advance. It is in the obtained category that the creative process is able to do the majority of its work.

Ritualized

The ritualized category is for various types of special eating occasions, such as social eating rituals, in which the individual does not necessarily specify the precise foods that will be eaten, but rather specifies participation in a specific eating ritual. The ritualized category allows for more spontaneous eating experiences that are tethered to a specific eating ritual (e.g., a meal at a restaurant, a wedding, etc.). Any number of ritualized eating occasions (including "none") can be specified for any specific day.

Obtained alternate plan

For any eating ritual that is specified in the ritualized category, the individual also includes an obtained alternate plan. The obtained alternate plan is the backup plan of the specific foods to be eaten in case the planned eating ritual falls through, for whatever reason.

Items in the obtained alternate plan are similar to items listed in the main "obtained" category: They are listed in specific amounts, and are obtained one day in advance.

It is not necessary to include items in all three categories (i.e., unlimited, obtained, and ritualized) on the plan for any given day. The key to success is to focus the majority of one's attention on the obtained category, as it is in this category that the creative process is able to carry out the majority of its work.

The most important thing to keep in mind is that in the ritual of bindling, the main task of the individual is simply to create and maintain the sacred space of self-mastery. While it is true that self-mastery is a powerful psychospiritual condition, the key to accessing its power is to always make it ridiculously easy to follow through with the designated plan.

This is the paradox of effortlessness. When the individual keeps the bindling process effortless, the psyche becomes increasingly disciplined on its own, without any pushing or pulling of the self.

4. After the items to be eaten on the Liminal Day have been selected, write out the selected plan on the Liminal Day form.

   Keep this as effortless as possible by using easily understood abbreviations and shorthand. Specific instructions for each of the three categories are as follows:

   Unlimited

   Write out the names of any foods to be permitted in unlimited amounts on the Liminal Day.

   Obtained

   Write out the (a) names and (b) specific amounts of foods designated to be eaten on the Liminal Day.

   Ritualized

   For any ritualized eating occasion, write out both (a) a description of the bounds of the eating occasion and (b) the obtained alternate plan, as follows:

Bounds of the eating occasion

Write out a specific description of the bounds of the eating occasion. The most simple way to do this is to write, "Whatever I wish to eat at . . .," and then specify the occasion.

Additional limitations and/or specifications may be included in the description, but it is important to not set oneself up for a situation in which one's intended plan might be compromised. For example, if an individual were to specify that exactly one plate of food is to be eaten at a particular social eating event, others who are present at the event may unknowingly compromise this person's plan by sampling from the person's plate, possibly even without asking for permission to do so.

The key to success is to chart out a path for oneself in which the follow-through is effortless and inevitable. Therefore, it is best to define the bounds of a ritualized eating occasion in such a way that the individual will be able to fully relax and enjoy the occasion, and rest assured that the plan is being carried out effortlessly and as intended.

243

Obtained alternate plan

After the description of the bounds of the eating occasion, write "Alt.:" followed by the (a) names and (b) specific amounts of foods designated to be eaten in case the eating occasion falls through, for whatever reason.

5. After the selected plan for the Liminal Day has been finalized and written out on the Liminal Day form, check off the OBT and DOC boxes on the Pre-Liminal Day form.

OBT box

Checking off the OBT box on the Pre-Liminal Day form indicates that all of the items listed as obtained on the Liminal Day form have been obtained.

This refers to both (a) items in the main obtained category and (b) items obtained as alternate (i.e., backup) for anything planned in the ritualized category.

DOC box

Checking off the DOC box on the Pre-Liminal Day form indicates that the full eating plan for the

244

Liminal Day has been documented (i.e., written out) on the Liminal Day form.

Optional

A series of Ws appears in the lower left-hand corner of the Pre-Liminal Day form and all subsequent forms. These Ws are provided for individuals who wish to track their water intake in whatever way is helpful to them.

LIMINAL DAY

The second day in the Three-Day Initiation Cycle is the Liminal Day.

The Liminal Day is a glowing day, and it glows in a complicated way.

The Liminal Day is a day of transition, a day that is neither this, nor that. On the Liminal Day, the initiate has departed from the everyday ordinary reality, but has not yet entered into the sacred space of self-mastery in its fullness.

The Liminal Day is an in-between space, a threshold, a place across which one passes.

The tasks completed on the Liminal Day are as follows:

1. Follow through with the eating plan specified on the Liminal Day form.

2. Write tomorrow's date in the lower right-hand corner of the Initiation Day form (i.e., the form on the page following the page on which the Liminal Day form appears).

3. Select a series of food items to be eaten on the Initiation Day, in the same way that the series of food items to be eaten on the Liminal Day was selected on the Pre-Liminal Day.

   Consider including some type of celebratory item to be enjoyed on the Initiation Day.

4. Write out the selected plan on the Initiation Day form, in the same way that the selected plan for the Liminal Day was written out on the Liminal Day form, on the Pre-Liminal Day.

   Make sure that all items listed as obtained have been obtained; this includes both (a) items in the main obtained category and (b) items obtained as alternate (i.e., backup) for anything planned in the ritualized category.

5. Check off the OBT and DOC boxes on the Liminal Day form.

On the Liminal Day

More than on any other day, the Liminal Day is a day on which it is very important to be gentle with oneself. The Liminal Day is a very special day given that the individual is transitioning from one experience of reality into another form of reality, i.e., into a specific type of sacred space. The individual is in the process of entering into this sacred space, but has not yet entered into it fully. At the same time, the individual is no longer in the ordinary everyday space of the day prior.

On the Liminal Day, the individual may at times feel out of sync or disconnected, as the individual has in fact disconnected from one experience of reality and is now transitioning into another form of reality.

At the same time, the Liminal Day is a day of magic and power. The individual may experience unusual synchronicities on this day. While feelings of unease may occur on the Liminal Day, underlying any such feelings is a deeper sense of magic, excitement, curiosity, and transformation.

The Liminal Day is a good day to clear out one's schedule and lay out some plans to do some fun, quiet, relaxing things that are enjoyable to the individual.

The Liminal Day is a day for the individual to acknowledge that a challenge is being introduced to the

248

self, and that a transition into a specific type of sacred space is in the process of occurring.

The Liminal Day is a day for the individual to do whatever it takes to soothe the self and ease the self through the day.

INITIATION DAY, or Day 1

The third and final day in the Three-Day Initiation Cycle is the Initiation Day.

On the Initiation Day, the individual wakes up having entered into the sacred space of self-mastery. The individual signifies this by writing the number "1" in the center of the laurel wreath at the top of the Initiation Day form.

This writing of the number "1" in the center of the laurel wreath is a deeply symbolic act. It is a designation of honor and an acknowledgement that the individual has entered into the sacred space of self-mastery.

On the Initiation Day, a sense of accomplishment gently ripples throughout the entire being of the initiate. It is highly adaptive to allow oneself to fully bask in the rippling sensations of this sense of accomplishment, this knowing that the individual has followed through with a designated, intended plan. To bask in this feeling is a high in and of itself, and at the same time, basking in this feeling energizes the ongoing bindling process and contributes to the sending out of ripple effects into all aspects of the life of the individual.

Also too, sometimes when we experience magic and transformation, the feelings of excitement may begin to feel overwhelming, and we may begin to feel afraid of the excitement. If the excitement gets to be too intense, this can be counterproductive. The key to success then is to allow oneself to feel excited about the success of the Initiation Day, and about the new possibilities and horizons that are opening up in one's life, and at the same time to keep oneself solidly, lightly grounded—that is, to just get on with the day. What we discover then is that it is actually in our embracing of the mundane that we discover the quiet, gentle moments that contain the true nectar of life.

So the first task then on the Initiation Day is simply to designate one's entry into the sacred space of self-mastery by writing the number "1" in the center of the laurel wreath at the top of the Initiation Day form.

The remaining tasks completed on the Initiation Day are essentially the same as the tasks completed on the Liminal Day:

1. Follow through with the eating plan specified on the Initiation Day (Day 1) form.

2. Write tomorrow's date in the lower right-hand corner of the Day 2 form (i.e., the form on the page following the page on which the Initiation Day form appears).

3. Select a series of food items to be eaten on Day 2, in the same way that food items were selected one day ahead on the previous two days.

4. Write out the selected plan on the Day 2 form, in the same way that the selected plans were written out one day ahead on the previous two days.

   Make sure that all items listed as obtained have been obtained, including both (a) items in the main obtained category and (b) items obtained as alternate (i.e., backup) for anything planned in the ritualized category.

5. Check off the OBT and DOC boxes on the Initiation Day (Day 1) form.

Day 2, Day 3, and on we go

The tasks completed on each ongoing day are as follows:

First, write the next consecutive day number ("2" on Day 2, "3" on Day 3, etc.) in the center of the laurel wreath at the top of the current day form (i.e., the form on which today's menu appears). This signifies continuation of the sacred space of self-mastery. Then,

1. Follow through with the eating plan as specified on the current day form.

2. Write tomorrow's date in the lower right-hand corner of the next day form (i.e., the form on the page following the page on which the current day form appears).

3. Select a series of food items to be eaten tomorrow, in the same way that food items were selected one day ahead on each day of the Three-Day Initiation Cycle.

253

4. Write out the selected plan on the next day form, in the same way that the selected plans were written out one day ahead on each day of the Three-Day Initiation Cycle.

   Make sure that all items listed as obtained have been obtained, including both (a) items in the main obtained category and (b) items obtained as alternate (i.e., backup) for anything planned in the ritualized category.

5. Check off the OBT and DOC boxes on the current day form.

The Daily Approach

Of the five daily bindling tasks listed above, task 1 — i.e., following through with today's menu — is something that can be spread across the entire day. On the current day form, the individual may wish to check off each specific food item as it is eaten throughout the course of the day.

To keep the daily process as effortless as possible, the individual may wish to complete tasks 2, 3, 4, and 5 as early as possible each day.

254

. . . and on we go

The individual who bindles gets to experience and enjoy the same sense of accomplishment experienced on the Initiation Day, each and every day thereafter, on an ongoing basis. Allowing oneself to fully enjoy this sense of accomplishment is highly adaptive in that it contributes to the desired outcome becoming materialized as quickly and as effectively as is possible.

At the same time, allowing one's psyche to become fully saturated in this ongoing sense of accomplishment and success is key to the ripple effects of bindling. Basking in the waves of accomplishment and success contributes to the rippling out of waves of accomplishment and success into all aspects of the life of the individual.

From here on out it's really just about having fun with the process, listening to the process, learning from it, and becoming one with it. The process refines itself and builds its own momentum as the individual maintains a stance of paradoxical detached attachment. With this stance, the individual focuses simply on going through the motions of the simple, few-minutes-daily bindling ritual, and then dwells entirely in one's desire for the outcome and in the multiple levels of ecstasy that are generated by the bindling ritual.

Priming the Pump

During the first little while after the Three-Day Initiation Cycle, the individual begins to develop a personal rhythm and begins to get into an effortless flow in the bindling process. This early stage of figuring out one's own personal effortless rhythm is similar to the process of priming a pump: The process begins with an initial challenge of bringing liquid into the pump, but then once it starts to flow, the process takes over and continues on its own, effortlessly.

If the bindling process ever feels too challenging during this initial stage of priming the pump—or at any point during the ongoing bindling process—then at that point the most important task of the individual is simply to scale back and do whatever it takes to keep the process as absolutely easy and effortless as is possible.

Then, at some point something magical happens. Something clicks. The pump becomes primed, and the process takes over and moves forward, seemingly of its own accord. The individual becomes caught up in a state of creative rapture and becomes as it were an observer of the creative process moving through the self.

At this point the individual gets to start having some fun with the evolving process. The individual begins to establish some basic patterns in the bindling process and begins to refine it as desired (see the How to Bindle chapter for guidance on this). The individual remains focused on dwelling entirely in ecstasy and desire, and meanwhile, the desired outcome begins to materialize on its own, gently, seemingly of its own accord.

Getting It Seamlessly Installed

Effortlessness is the most important ingredient of success in the ongoing bindling process. When a process is effortless, it is impossible for anything to get in its way.

To fully facilitate the effortlessness of the bindling process, the individual may wish to consider the use of a simple calendar and/or a reminder object, as a way of reminding oneself to complete the daily bindling tasks.

When an item such as a calendar or a reminder object is used by the individual, this item serves as an annex of the individual's brain, an annex that takes care of the remembering work on the individual's behalf, so that the individual can let go of it completely.

Through the use of a calendar and/or a reminder object, the individual becomes able to completely let go of any need to think about bindling except during the few minutes per day during which the individual is deliberately focused on completing the daily bindling ritual.

Then, if thoughts about bindling do occur at other times during the day, they aren't self-tugging thoughts such as, "Oh, I need to remember to . . . ." Rather, they are inspired reflections

257

about how to refine one's ongoing bindling process, ideas for the daily menu, and so on.

Neither the use of a calendar nor the use of a reminder object is required for successful bindling. Rather, these are simply strategies that are available to the individual, one or both of which the individual may choose to implement for the purpose of getting bindling seamlessly installed into one's daily routine.

Getting bindling seamlessly installed into one's daily routine frees up the psyche so that it is able to enter into the deepest possible communion with the creative process. It makes it possible for the individual to empty the mind completely, and to thereby become fully receptive to the full resplendence of life.

Use of a calendar (optional)

A simple way of using a calendar to remind oneself to complete the daily bindling tasks is to write down on the calendar for today the notation "BI, E :||D". This notation consists of the following components:

BI = Bindle

> This refers to all of the daily bindling tasks except for following through with the eating plan specified on the current day form.

258

After all bindling tasks (except for eating today's food) have been completed, the individual crosses out the "BI" on today's calendar (i.e., "B̶I̶").

E = Eat

This refers to following through with the eating plan specified on the current day form.

This is separated out from "BI" because it is best to get all the other daily bindling tasks completed as early as possible, whereas the enjoyment of today's food is likely to extend across the entire duration of the day.

After the individual has followed through with the eating plan specified for today, the individual crosses out the "E" on today's calendar (i.e., "E̶").

:‖D = Repeat notation for next day

This refers, simply, to writing the "BI, E :‖D" notation on the calendar for the following day. In other words, it refers to the literal act of writing "BI, E :‖D" on the calendar for the following day.

After the individual has written "BI, E :‖D" on the calendar for the following day, the individual crosses out the ":‖D" on today's calendar (i.e., ":̶‖̶D̶").

Using the ":‖D" symbol is a way of keeping the bindling process grounded in the moment, i.e., by keeping it grounded in the current day-night-day cycle. There is never any need to write down the daily "BI, E :‖D" notation more than one day in advance.

On most days, the individual is likely to complete the "BI" and the ":‖D" tasks earlier in the day, and to complete the "E" task later in the day. Therefore, the daily notation is likely to develop as follows:

At the beginning of the day, the notation appears as "BI, E :‖D".

Then, whenever the individual gets to it (the sooner the better), the individual (a) completes the daily bindling tasks (except eating today's food) and (b) writes the notation "BI, E :‖D" on the calendar for tomorrow. To indicate that these two tasks have been completed, the individual then crosses out the "BI" and the ":‖D" on the calendar for today. Now the notation appears as "B̶I̶, E :̶‖̶D̶".

Then, after the individual has followed through with the eating plan specified for today (most likely towards the end of the day), the individual then crosses out the "E" on the calendar for today. The notation then appears as "B̶I̶,̶ E̶ :̶‖̶D̶". At this point, all items are crossed off in the notation.

Use of a reminder object (optional)

A reminder object is simply an object the individual places near the individual's bed, to remind the individual to complete the daily bindling tasks before going to bed.

A reminder object is used as follows:

The individual places the reminder object in a location in which the individual will be forced to move the object in order to be able to get into bed. In this way, the individual is reminded to complete all bindling tasks for today before going to bed.

After the individual has completed all bindling tasks for the day and is now ready to go to bed, the individual then moves the object away from the bed and places it in a location in which the individual will be forced to move it again in the morning. In other words, the individual places the object in such a way that in the morning, the individual will be forced to move the object back to its daytime location near the bed, before the individual will be able to proceed with the individual's morning routine.

So then when the individual wakes up in the morning and gets out of bed, the individual moves the reminder object back to its daytime location near the bed, so that the individual will again that night be forced to move the object out of the way before getting into bed.

261

A reminder object reminds the individual to complete the daily bindling tasks prior to the end of each day. Of course, it is almost always best to complete the daily bindling tasks earlier rather than later, but either way, having a reminder object near one's bed provides the individual with a gentle reminder to complete the daily bindling tasks prior to the end of the day. In this way, the individual becomes free to empty the mind fully and to enter into the deepest possible communion with the creative process.

PRE-LIMINAL DAY

OBT	DOC

w w w w w w w w

Y Y M M D D

_ _ _ _ _ _

LIMINAL DAY

OBT	DOC

Unlimited

Obtained ITEMS AND AMOUNTS

Ritualized
INCL OBTAINED ALT PLAN

W W W W W W W W

Y Y M M D D

‗ ‗ ‗ ‗ ‗ ‗

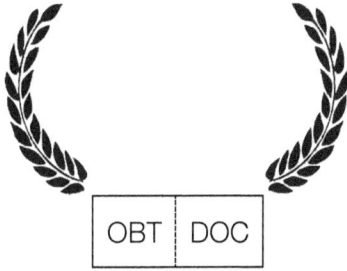

OBT | DOC

Unlimited

Obtained ITEMS AND AMOUNTS

Ritualized
INCL OBTAINED ALT PLAN

Y Y M M D D

W W W W W W W W W   __ __ __ __ __ __

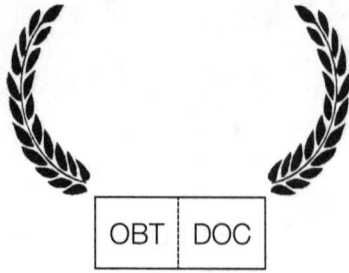

OBT | DOC

Unlimited

Obtained ITEMS AND AMOUNTS

Ritualized
INCL OBTAINED ALT PLAN

W W W W W W W W

Y Y M M D D
__ __ __ __ __ __

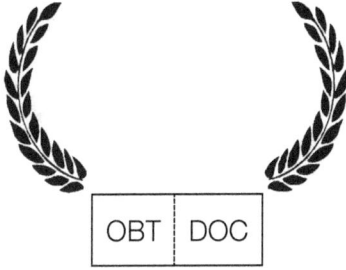

| OBT | DOC |

Unlimited

Obtained ITEMS AND AMOUNTS

Ritualized
INCL OBTAINED ALT PLAN

W   W   W   W   W   W   W   W

Y   Y   M   M   D   D

___   ___   ___   ___   ___   ___

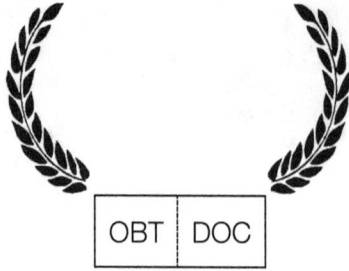

OBT | DOC

Unlimited

Obtained ITEMS AND AMOUNTS

Ritualized
INCL OBTAINED ALT PLAN

W   W   W   W   W   W   W   W

Y   Y   M   M   D   D

___ ___ ___ ___ ___ ___

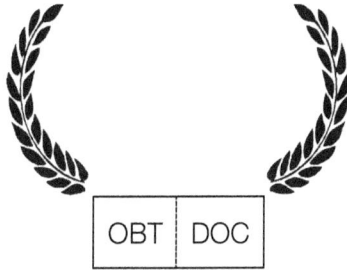

OBT | DOC

Unlimited

Obtained ITEMS AND AMOUNTS

Ritualized
INCL OBTAINED ALT PLAN

Y Y M M D D

W W W W W W W W   __ __ __ __ __ __

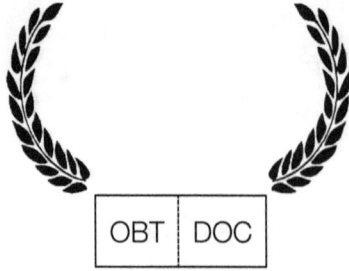

OBT | DOC

Unlimited

Obtained ITEMS AND AMOUNTS

Ritualized
INCL OBTAINED ALT PLAN

W W W W W W W W

Y Y M M D D
___ ___ ___ ___ ___ ___

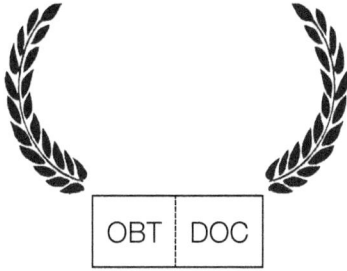

OBT | DOC

Unlimited

Obtained ITEMS AND AMOUNTS

Ritualized
INCL OBTAINED ALT PLAN

W W W W W W W W W

Y Y M M D D

___ ___ ___ ___ ___ ___

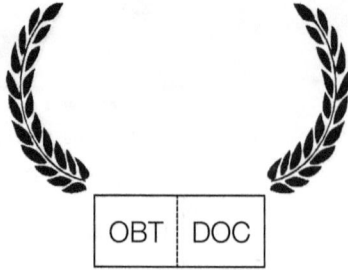

OBT | DOC

Unlimited

Obtained ITEMS AND AMOUNTS

Ritualized
INCL OBTAINED ALT PLAN

W W W W W W W W

Y Y M M D D

___ ___ ___ ___ ___ ___

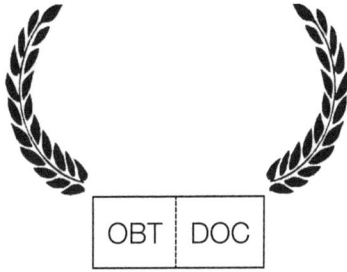

OBT | DOC

Unlimited

Obtained ITEMS AND AMOUNTS

Ritualized
INCL OBTAINED ALT PLAN

Y Y M M D D

W W W W W W W W   __ __ __ __ __ __

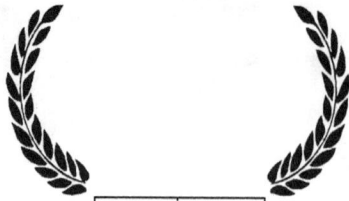

OBT	DOC

Unlimited

Obtained ITEMS AND AMOUNTS

Ritualized
INCL OBTAINED ALT PLAN

W   W   W   W   W   W   W   W

Y   Y   M   M   D   D

___   ___   ___   ___   ___   ___

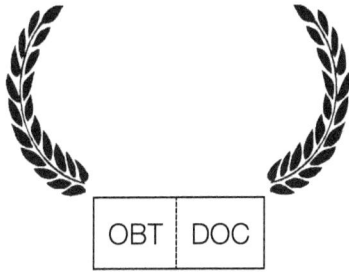

| OBT | DOC |

Unlimited

Obtained ITEMS AND AMOUNTS

Ritualized
INCL OBTAINED ALT PLAN

Y Y M M D D

W W W W W W W W   __ __ __ __ __ __

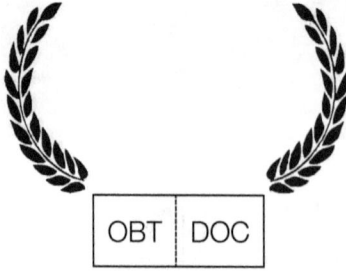

OBT	DOC

Unlimited

Obtained ITEMS AND AMOUNTS

Ritualized
INCL OBTAINED ALT PLAN

W W W W W W W W W

Y Y M M D D
__ __ __ __ __ __

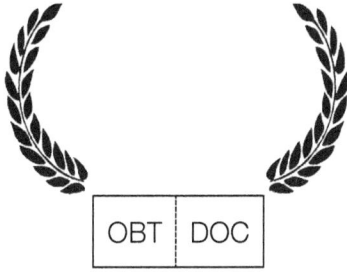

| OBT | DOC |

Unlimited

Obtained ITEMS AND AMOUNTS

Ritualized
INCL OBTAINED ALT PLAN

W   W   W   W   W   W   W   W

Y   Y   M   M   D   D

__   __   __   __   __   __

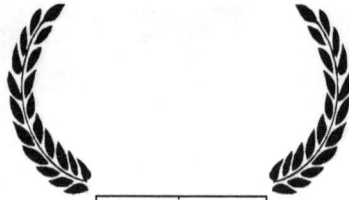

OBT	DOC

Unlimited

Obtained ITEMS AND AMOUNTS

Ritualized
INCL OBTAINED ALT PLAN

W   W   W   W   W   W   W   W   W

Y   Y   M   M   D   D

_   _   _   _   _   _

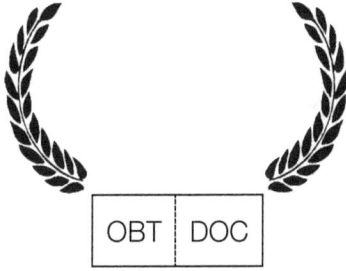

OBT | DOC

Unlimited

Obtained ITEMS AND AMOUNTS

Ritualized
INCL OBTAINED ALT PLAN

W W W W W W W W W

Y Y M M D D
__ __ __ __ __ __

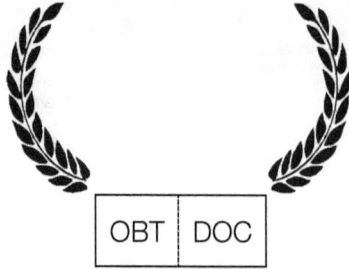

OBT	DOC

Unlimited

Obtained ITEMS AND AMOUNTS

Ritualized
INCL OBTAINED ALT PLAN

W   W   W   W   W   W   W   W

Y   Y   M   M   D   D

—   —   —   —   —   —

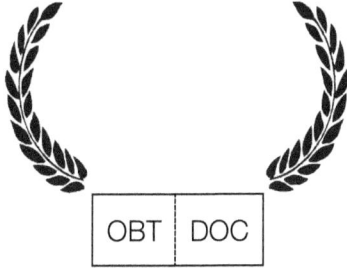

OBT | DOC

Unlimited

Obtained ITEMS AND AMOUNTS

Ritualized
INCL OBTAINED ALT PLAN

W W W W W W W W

Y Y M M D D

_ _ _ _ _ _

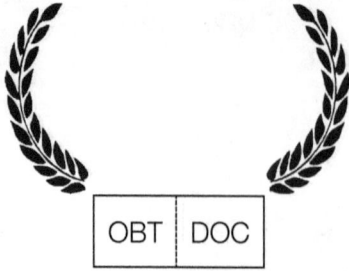

OBT	DOC

Unlimited

Obtained ITEMS AND AMOUNTS

Ritualized
INCL OBTAINED ALT PLAN

W   W   W   W   W   W   W   W   W

Y   Y   M   M   D   D

___   ___   ___   ___   ___   ___

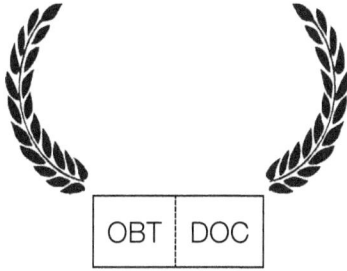

OBT | DOC

Unlimited

Obtained ITEMS AND AMOUNTS

Ritualized
INCL OBTAINED ALT PLAN

Y Y M M D D

W W W W W W W W W

__ __ __ __ __ __

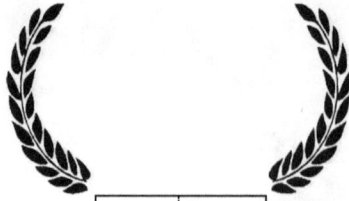

OBT	DOC

Unlimited

Obtained ITEMS AND AMOUNTS

Ritualized
INCL OBTAINED ALT PLAN

Y Y M M D D
_ _ _ _ _ _

W W W W W W W W

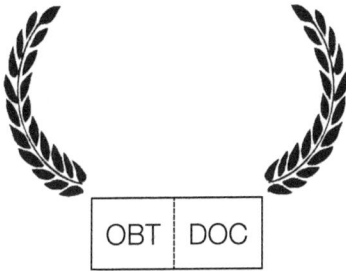

OBT	DOC

Unlimited

Obtained ITEMS AND AMOUNTS

Ritualized
INCL OBTAINED ALT PLAN

W   W   W   W   W   W   W   W   W

Y   Y   M   M   D   D

___   ___   ___   ___   ___   ___

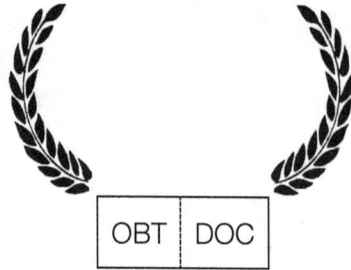

OBT | DOC

Unlimited

Obtained ITEMS AND AMOUNTS

Ritualized
INCL OBTAINED ALT PLAN

W W W W W W W W

Y Y M M D D
_ _ _ _ _ _

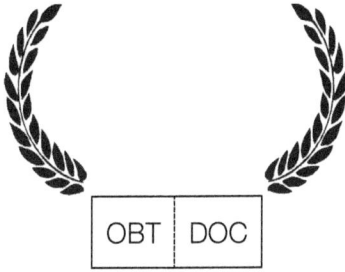

OBT | DOC

Unlimited

Obtained ITEMS AND AMOUNTS

Ritualized
INCL OBTAINED ALT PLAN

Y   Y   M   M   D   D

W   W   W   W   W   W   W   W   __   __   __   __   __   __

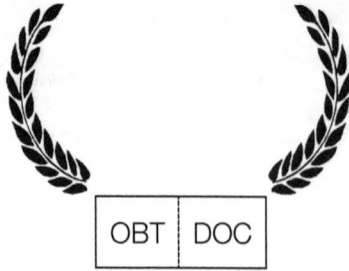

OBT	DOC

Unlimited

Obtained ITEMS AND AMOUNTS

Ritualized
INCL OBTAINED ALT PLAN

W W W W W W W W

Y Y M M D D

_ _ _ _ _ _

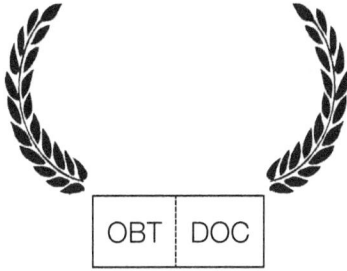

OBT | DOC

Unlimited

Obtained ITEMS AND AMOUNTS

Ritualized
INCL OBTAINED ALT PLAN

Y Y M M D D

W W W W W W W W   __ __ __ __ __ __

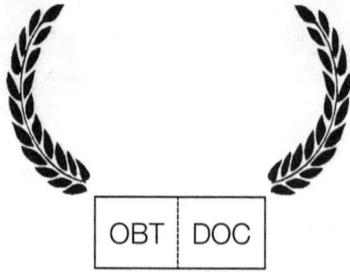

OBT	DOC

Unlimited

Obtained ITEMS AND AMOUNTS

Ritualized
INCL OBTAINED ALT PLAN

W W W W W W W W W

Y Y M M D D

_ _ _ _ _ _

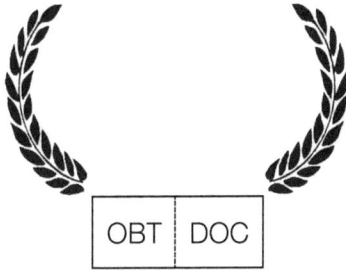

OBT | DOC

Unlimited

Obtained ITEMS AND AMOUNTS

Ritualized
INCL OBTAINED ALT PLAN

W W W W W W W W W

Y   Y   M   M   D   D

__ __ __ __ __ __

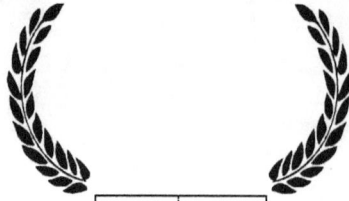

OBT	DOC

Unlimited

Obtained ITEMS AND AMOUNTS

Ritualized
INCL OBTAINED ALT PLAN

W   W   W   W   W   W   W   W

Y   Y   M   M   D   D

—   —   —   —   —   —

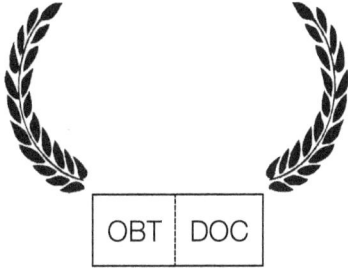

OBT	DOC

Unlimited

Obtained ITEMS AND AMOUNTS

Ritualized
INCL OBTAINED ALT PLAN

W W W W W W W W W

Y Y M M D D

__ __ __ __ __ __

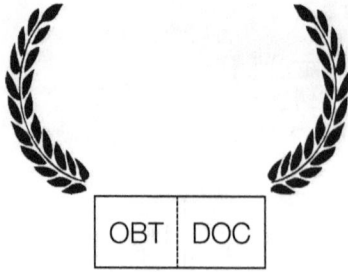

OBT	DOC

Unlimited

Obtained ITEMS AND AMOUNTS

Ritualized
INCL OBTAINED ALT PLAN

W   W   W   W   W   W   W   W

Y   Y   M   M   D   D

___   ___   ___   ___   ___   ___

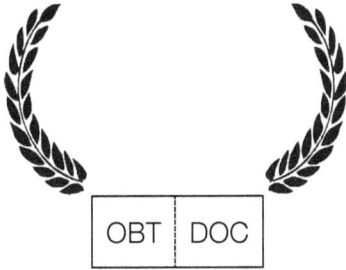

OBT	DOC

Unlimited

Obtained ITEMS AND AMOUNTS

Ritualized
INCL OBTAINED ALT PLAN

w w w w w w w w

Y Y M M D D

__ __ __ __ __ __

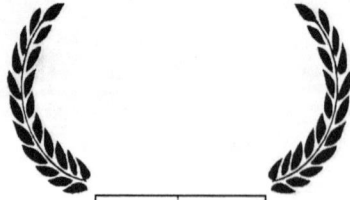

OBT	DOC

Unlimited

Obtained ITEMS AND AMOUNTS

Ritualized
INCL OBTAINED ALT PLAN

W W W W W W W W W

Y Y M M D D

— — — — — —

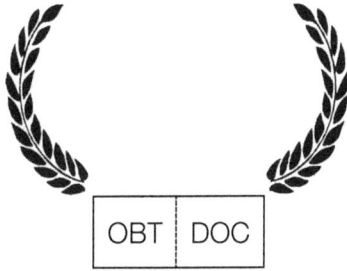

OBT | DOC

Unlimited

Obtained ITEMS AND AMOUNTS

Ritualized
INCL OBTAINED ALT PLAN

Y Y M M D D

W W W W W W W W   __ __ __ __ __ __

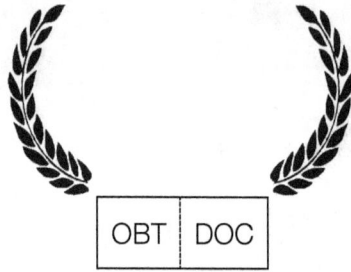

OBT | DOC

Unlimited

Obtained ITEMS AND AMOUNTS

Ritualized
INCL OBTAINED ALT PLAN

W W W W W W W W

Y Y M M D D

— — — — — —

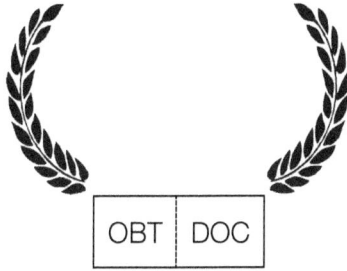

OBT | DOC

Unlimited

Obtained ITEMS AND AMOUNTS

Ritualized
INCL OBTAINED ALT PLAN

W W W W W W W W

Y Y M M D D

__ __ __ __ __ __

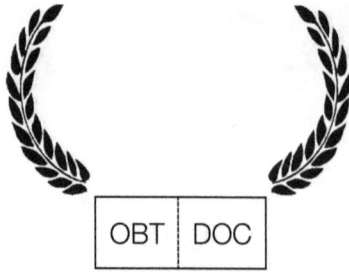

OBT	DOC

Unlimited

Obtained ITEMS AND AMOUNTS

Ritualized
INCL OBTAINED ALT PLAN

W W W W W W W W W

Y Y M M D D

— — — — — —

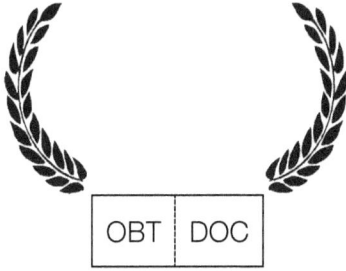

OBT | DOC

Unlimited

Obtained ITEMS AND AMOUNTS

Ritualized
INCL OBTAINED ALT PLAN

W W W W W W W W

Y Y M M D D

__ __ __ __ __ __

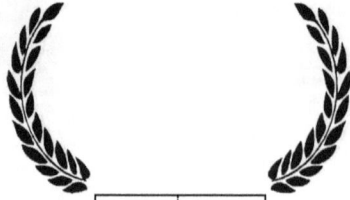

OBT | DOC

Unlimited

Obtained ITEMS AND AMOUNTS

Ritualized
INCL OBTAINED ALT PLAN

W   W   W   W   W   W   W   W

Y   Y   M   M   D   D

—   —   —   —   —   —

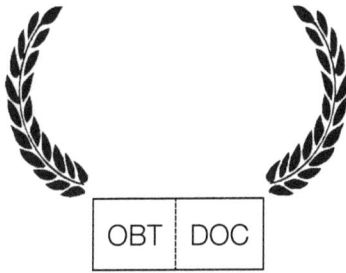

OBT	DOC

Unlimited

Obtained ITEMS AND AMOUNTS

Ritualized
INCL OBTAINED ALT PLAN

W W W W W W W W W

Y   Y   M   M   D   D

__ __ __ __ __ __

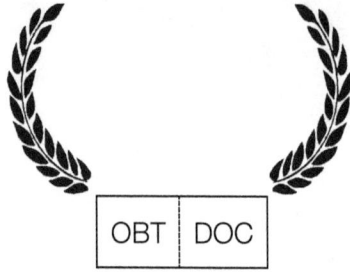

OBT | DOC

Unlimited

Obtained ITEMS AND AMOUNTS

Ritualized
INCL OBTAINED ALT PLAN

W   W   W   W   W   W   W   W

Y   Y   M   M   D   D

—   —   —   —   —   —

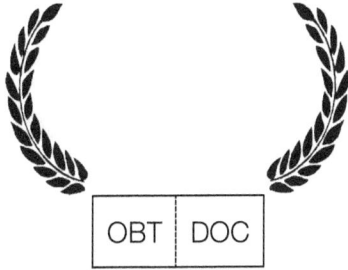

OBT | DOC

Unlimited

Obtained ITEMS AND AMOUNTS

Ritualized
INCL OBTAINED ALT PLAN

Y Y M M D D

w w w w w w w w w   __ __ __ __ __ __

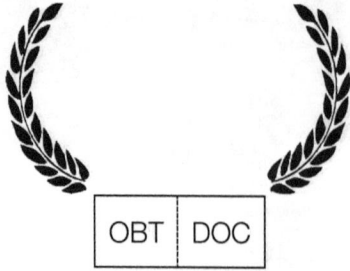

OBT	DOC

Unlimited

Obtained ITEMS AND AMOUNTS

Ritualized
INCL OBTAINED ALT PLAN

W W W W W W W W

Y Y M M D D

— — — — — —

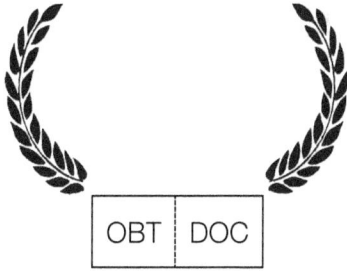

OBT | DOC

Unlimited

Obtained ITEMS AND AMOUNTS

Ritualized
INCL OBTAINED ALT PLAN

W W W W W W W W

Y Y M M D D

__ __ __ __ __ __

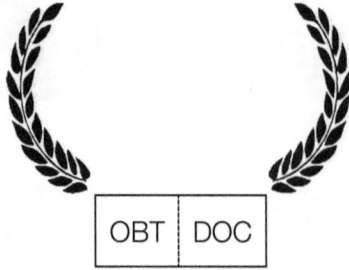

OBT	DOC

Unlimited

Obtained ITEMS AND AMOUNTS

Ritualized
INCL OBTAINED ALT PLAN

W   W   W   W   W   W   W   W

Y   Y   M   M   D   D

—   —   —   —   —   —

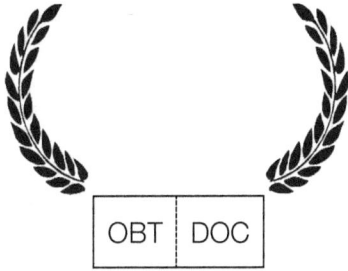

OBT | DOC

Unlimited

Obtained ITEMS AND AMOUNTS

Ritualized
INCL OBTAINED ALT PLAN

W W W W W W W W W

Y Y M M D D

__ __ __ __ __ __

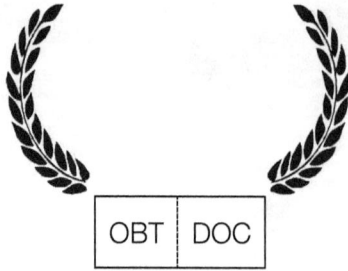

OBT	DOC

Unlimited

Obtained ITEMS AND AMOUNTS

Ritualized
INCL OBTAINED ALT PLAN

W W W W W W W W

Y Y M M D D

___ ___ ___ ___ ___ ___

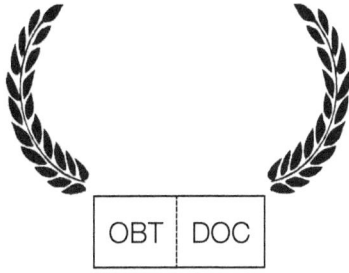

OBT | DOC

Unlimited

Obtained ITEMS AND AMOUNTS

Ritualized
INCL OBTAINED ALT PLAN

W   W   W   W   W   W   W   W

Y   Y   M   M   D   D

__ __ __ __ __ __

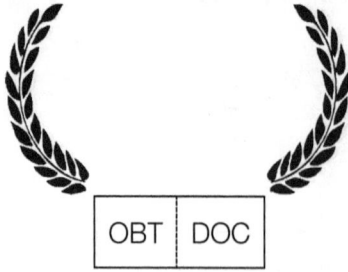

OBT	DOC

Unlimited

Obtained ITEMS AND AMOUNTS

Ritualized
INCL OBTAINED ALT PLAN

W W W W W W W W W

Y Y M M D D

_ _ _ _ _ _

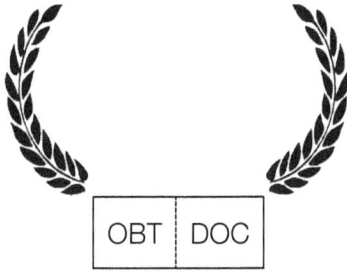

OBT | DOC

Unlimited

Obtained ITEMS AND AMOUNTS

Ritualized
INCL OBTAINED ALT PLAN

Y Y M M D D

W W W W W W W W   __ __ __ __ __ __

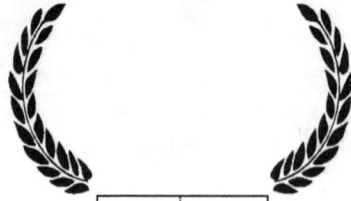

OBT | DOC

Unlimited

Obtained ITEMS AND AMOUNTS

Ritualized
INCL OBTAINED ALT PLAN

W W W W W W W W

Y Y M M D D
_ _ _ _ _ _

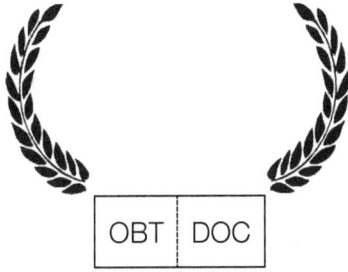

OBT | DOC

Unlimited

Obtained ITEMS AND AMOUNTS

Ritualized
INCL OBTAINED ALT PLAN

W W W W W W W W W

Y Y M M D D

__ __ __ __ __ __

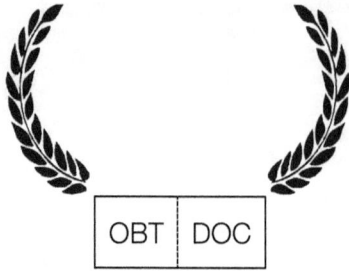

OBT | DOC

Unlimited

Obtained ITEMS AND AMOUNTS

Ritualized
INCL OBTAINED ALT PLAN

W W W W W W W W W

Y Y M M D D
— — — — — —

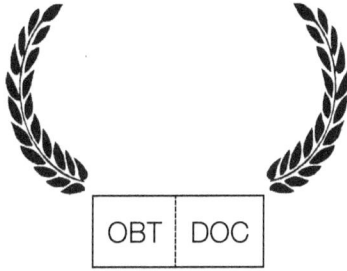

```
OBT | DOC
```

Unlimited

Obtained ITEMS AND AMOUNTS

Ritualized
INCL OBTAINED ALT PLAN

Y Y M M D D

w w w w w w w w   __ __ __ __ __ __

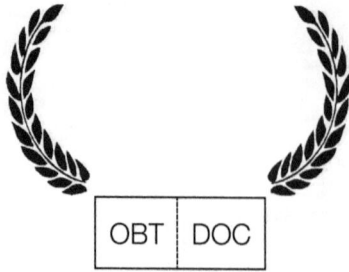

OBT	DOC

Unlimited

Obtained ITEMS AND AMOUNTS

Ritualized
INCL OBTAINED ALT PLAN

W W W W W W W W W

Y Y M M D D
— — — — — —

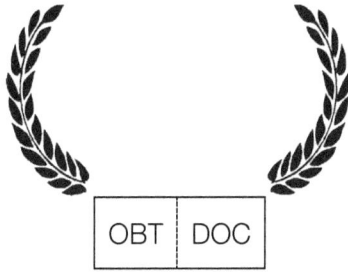

OBT | DOC

Unlimited

Obtained ITEMS AND AMOUNTS

Ritualized
INCL OBTAINED ALT PLAN

W W W W W W W W

Y Y M M D D
_ _ _ _ _ _

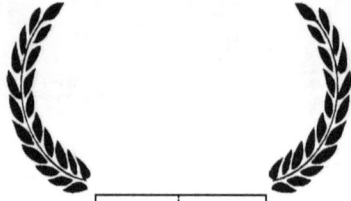

OBT | DOC

Unlimited

Obtained ITEMS AND AMOUNTS

Ritualized
INCL OBTAINED ALT PLAN

W W W W W W W W

Y Y M M D D
_ _ _ _ _ _

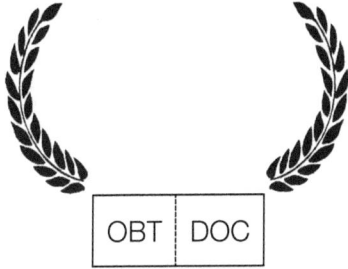

OBT | DOC

Unlimited

Obtained ITEMS AND AMOUNTS

Ritualized
INCL OBTAINED ALT PLAN

Y Y M M D D

w w w w w w w w   __ __ __ __ __ __

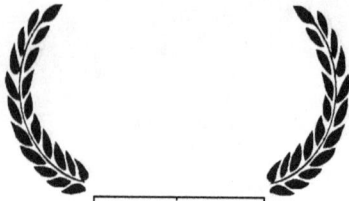

OBT	DOC

Unlimited

Obtained ITEMS AND AMOUNTS

Ritualized
INCL OBTAINED ALT PLAN

W W W W W W W W W

Y	Y	M	M	D	D
—	—	—	—	—	—

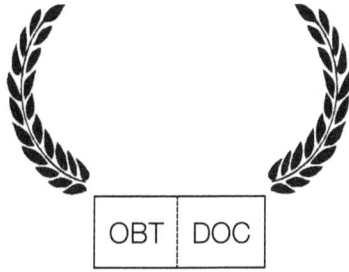

OBT	DOC

Unlimited

Obtained ITEMS AND AMOUNTS

Ritualized
INCL OBTAINED ALT PLAN

Y   Y   M   M   D   D

W   W   W   W   W   W   W   W   __ __ __ __ __ __

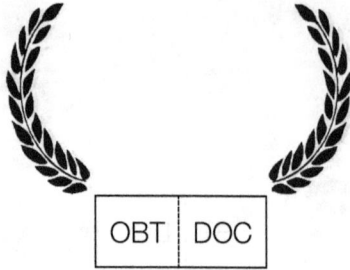

OBT	DOC

Unlimited

Obtained ITEMS AND AMOUNTS

Ritualized
INCL OBTAINED ALT PLAN

W W W W W W W W

Y Y M M D D
— — — — — —

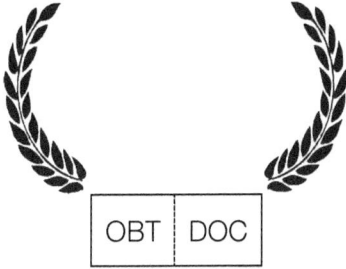

OBT | DOC

Unlimited

Obtained ITEMS AND AMOUNTS

Ritualized
INCL OBTAINED ALT PLAN

W W W W W W W W W

Y Y M M D D

___ ___ ___ ___ ___ ___

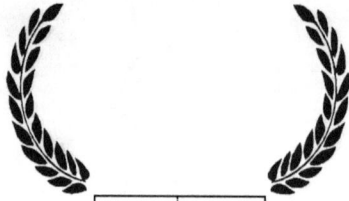

OBT | DOC

Unlimited

Obtained ITEMS AND AMOUNTS

Ritualized
INCL OBTAINED ALT PLAN

W W W W W W W W

Y Y M M D D
_ _ _ _ _ _

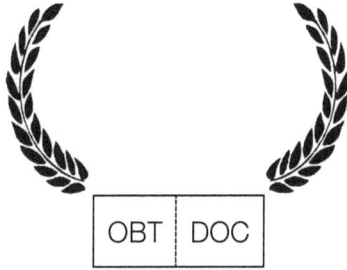

OBT	DOC

Unlimited

Obtained ITEMS AND AMOUNTS

Ritualized
INCL OBTAINED ALT PLAN

W   W   W   W   W   W   W   W

Y   Y   M   M   D   D

__   __   __   __   __   __

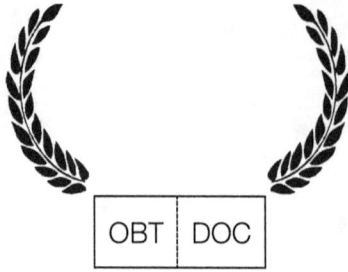

OBT | DOC

Unlimited

Obtained ITEMS AND AMOUNTS

Ritualized
INCL OBTAINED ALT PLAN

W W W W W W W W

Y Y M M D D
— — — — — —

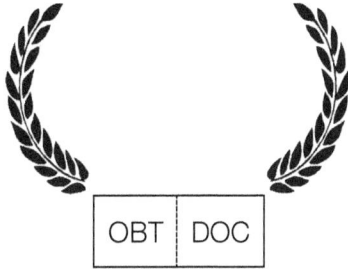

OBT	DOC

Unlimited

Obtained ITEMS AND AMOUNTS

Ritualized
INCL OBTAINED ALT PLAN

W W W W W W W W

Y Y M M D D

__ __ __ __ __ __

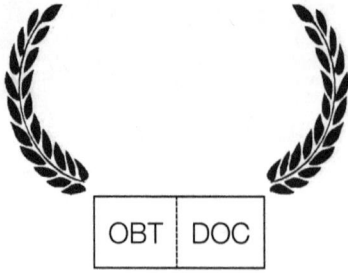

| OBT | DOC |

Unlimited

Obtained ITEMS AND AMOUNTS

Ritualized
INCL OBTAINED ALT PLAN

W   W   W   W   W   W   W   W

Y   Y   M   M   D   D
___   ___   ___   ___   ___   ___

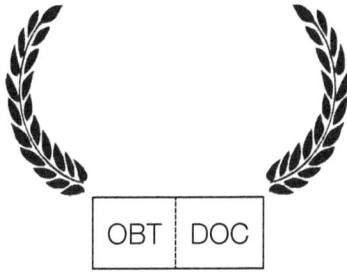

OBT | DOC

Unlimited

Obtained ITEMS AND AMOUNTS

Ritualized
INCL OBTAINED ALT PLAN

W W W W W W W W

Y Y M M D D
_ _ _ _ _ _

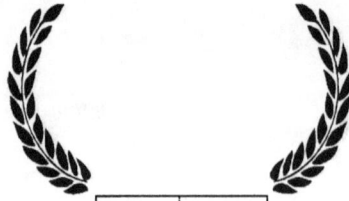

| OBT | DOC |

Unlimited

Obtained ITEMS AND AMOUNTS

Ritualized
INCL OBTAINED ALT PLAN

W W W W W W W W W

Y Y M M D D

_ _ _ _ _ _

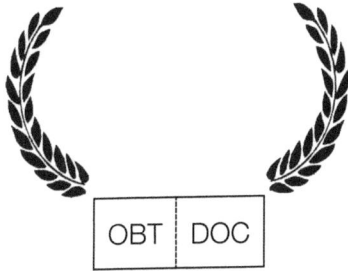

OBT	DOC

Unlimited

Obtained ITEMS AND AMOUNTS

Ritualized
INCL OBTAINED ALT PLAN

Y Y M M D D

w w w w w w w w   __ __ __ __ __ __

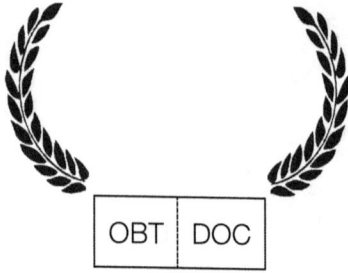

OBT	DOC

Unlimited

Obtained ITEMS AND AMOUNTS

Ritualized
INCL OBTAINED ALT PLAN

W   W   W   W   W   W   W   W

Y   Y   M   M   D   D

—   —   —   —   —   —

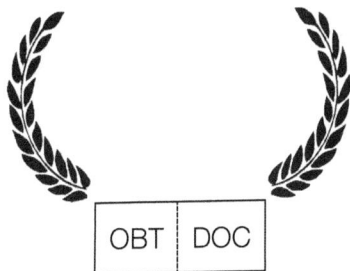

OBT	DOC

Unlimited

Obtained ITEMS AND AMOUNTS

Ritualized
INCL OBTAINED ALT PLAN

W W W W W W W W

Y   Y   M   M   D   D

___ ___ ___ ___ ___ ___

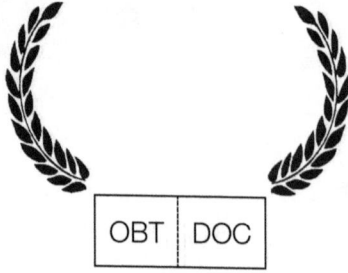

OBT | DOC

Unlimited

Obtained ITEMS AND AMOUNTS

Ritualized
INCL OBTAINED ALT PLAN

W W W W W W W W

Y Y M M D D
_ _ _ _ _ _

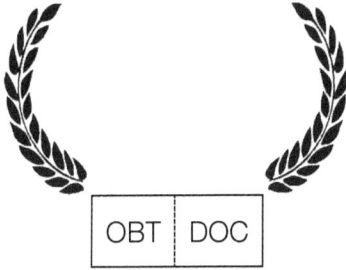

OBT | DOC

Unlimited

Obtained ITEMS AND AMOUNTS

Ritualized
INCL OBTAINED ALT PLAN

Y   Y   M   M   D   D

w   w   w   w   w   w   w   w   __ __ __ __ __ __

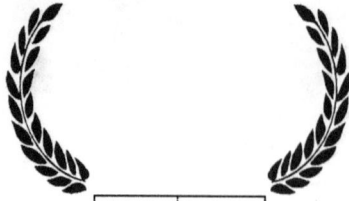

OBT | DOC

Unlimited

Obtained ITEMS AND AMOUNTS

Ritualized
INCL OBTAINED ALT PLAN

W   W   W   W   W   W   W   W

Y   Y   M   M   D   D

___ ___ ___ ___ ___ ___

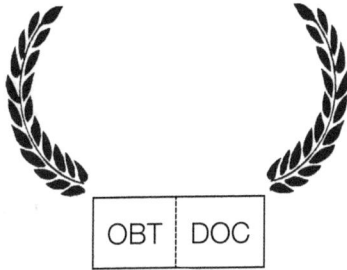

OBT | DOC

Unlimited

Obtained ITEMS AND AMOUNTS

Ritualized
INCL OBTAINED ALT PLAN

Y   Y   M   M   D   D

w w w w w w w w   __ __ __ __ __ __

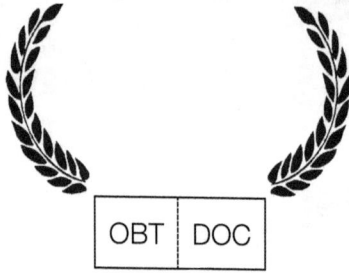

OBT | DOC

Unlimited

Obtained ITEMS AND AMOUNTS

Ritualized
INCL OBTAINED ALT PLAN

W W W W W W W W W

Y   Y   M   M   D   D

—   —   —   —   —   —

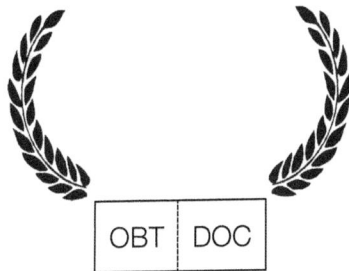

OBT	DOC

Unlimited

Obtained ITEMS AND AMOUNTS

Ritualized
INCL OBTAINED ALT PLAN

			Y	Y	M	M	D	D
w w w w w w w w			__	__	__	__	__	__

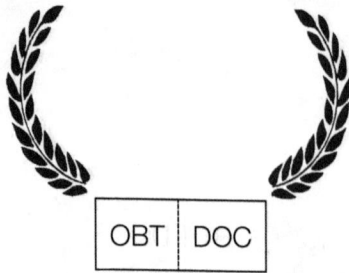

OBT	DOC

Unlimited

Obtained ITEMS AND AMOUNTS

Ritualized
INCL OBTAINED ALT PLAN

W W W W W W W W

Y Y M M D D

— — — — — —

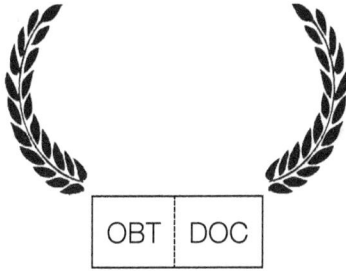

OBT | DOC

Unlimited

Obtained ITEMS AND AMOUNTS

Ritualized
INCL OBTAINED ALT PLAN

Y Y M M D D

W W W W W W W W W   __ __ __ __ __ __

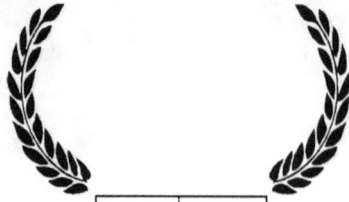

OBT | DOC

Unlimited

Obtained ITEMS AND AMOUNTS

Ritualized
INCL OBTAINED ALT PLAN

W W W W W W W W W

Y Y M M D D

_ _ _ _ _ _

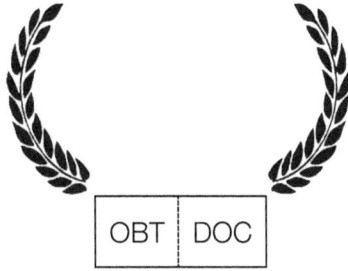

OBT	DOC

Unlimited

Obtained ITEMS AND AMOUNTS

Ritualized
INCL OBTAINED ALT PLAN

W W W W W W W W

Y Y M M D D

— — — — — —

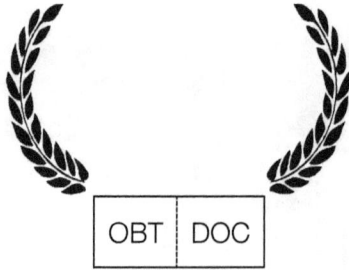

OBT | DOC

Unlimited

Obtained ITEMS AND AMOUNTS

Ritualized
INCL OBTAINED ALT PLAN

Y Y M M D D

W W W W W W W W   _ _ _ _ _ _

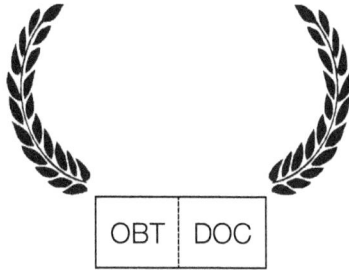

OBT	DOC

Unlimited

Obtained ITEMS AND AMOUNTS

Ritualized
INCL OBTAINED ALT PLAN

W W W W W W W W

Y Y M M D D

___ ___ ___ ___ ___ ___

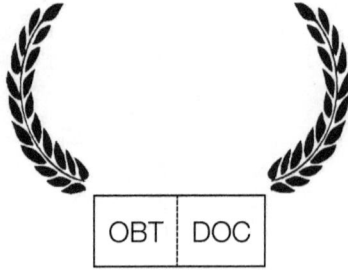

OBT | DOC

Unlimited

Obtained ITEMS AND AMOUNTS

Ritualized
INCL OBTAINED ALT PLAN

Y Y M M D D

W W W W W W W W W   __ __ __ __ __ __

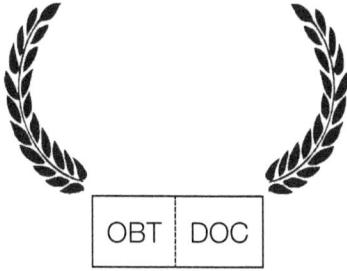

OBT	DOC

Unlimited

Obtained ITEMS AND AMOUNTS

Ritualized
INCL OBTAINED ALT PLAN

W W W W W W W W

Y Y M M D D

— — — — — —

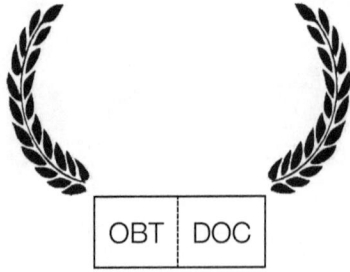

OBT | DOC

Unlimited

Obtained ITEMS AND AMOUNTS

Ritualized
INCL OBTAINED ALT PLAN

W W W W W W W W

Y   Y   M   M   D   D
__ __ __ __ __ __

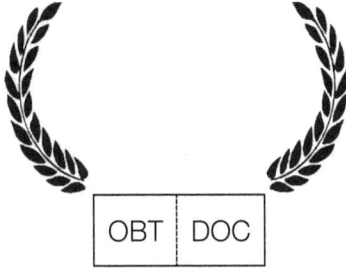

OBT | DOC

Unlimited

Obtained ITEMS AND AMOUNTS

Ritualized
INCL OBTAINED ALT PLAN

Y Y M M D D

W W W W W W W W   __ __ __ __ __ __

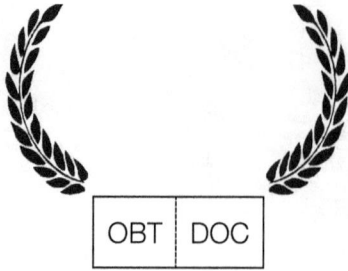

OBT | DOC

Unlimited

Obtained ITEMS AND AMOUNTS

Ritualized
INCL OBTAINED ALT PLAN

Y Y M M D D

W W W W W W W W   __ __ __ __ __ __

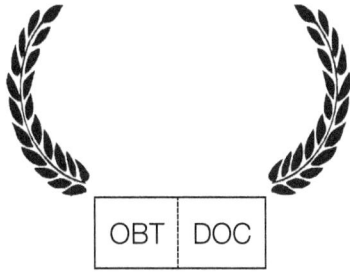

OBT	DOC

Unlimited

Obtained ITEMS AND AMOUNTS

Ritualized
INCL OBTAINED ALT PLAN

W W W W W W W W

Y Y M M D D

__ __ __ __ __ __

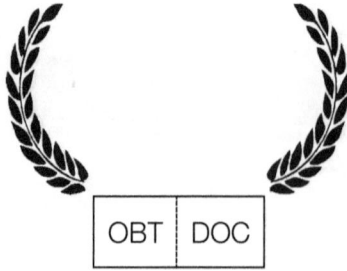

OBT	DOC

Unlimited

Obtained ITEMS AND AMOUNTS

Ritualized
INCL OBTAINED ALT PLAN

Y Y M M D D

W W W W W W W W __ __ __ __ __ __

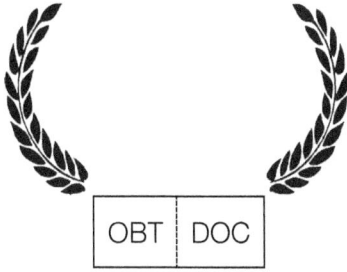

OBT | DOC

Unlimited

Obtained ITEMS AND AMOUNTS

Ritualized
INCL OBTAINED ALT PLAN

W W W W W W W W

Y Y M M D D

_ _ _ _ _ _

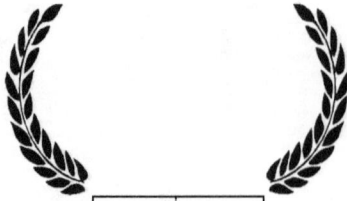

OBT	DOC

Unlimited

Obtained ITEMS AND AMOUNTS

Ritualized
INCL OBTAINED ALT PLAN

W W W W W W W W

Y Y M M D D

_ _ _ _ _ _

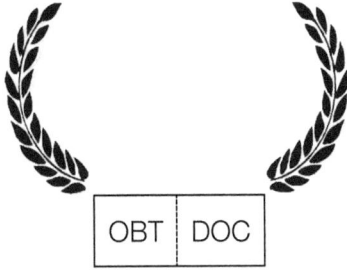

OBT	DOC

Unlimited

Obtained ITEMS AND AMOUNTS

Ritualized
INCL OBTAINED ALT PLAN

W   W   W   W   W   W   W   W

Y   Y   M   M   D   D

___   ___   ___   ___   ___   ___

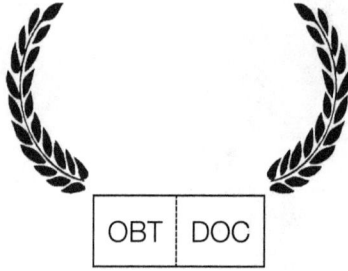

OBT | DOC

Unlimited

Obtained ITEMS AND AMOUNTS

Ritualized
INCL OBTAINED ALT PLAN

Y Y M M D D

W W W W W W W W   __ __ __ __ __ __

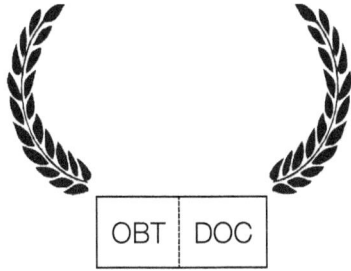

OBT | DOC

Unlimited

Obtained ITEMS AND AMOUNTS

Ritualized
INCL OBTAINED ALT PLAN

W W W W W W W W W

Y Y M M D D

__ __ __ __ __ __

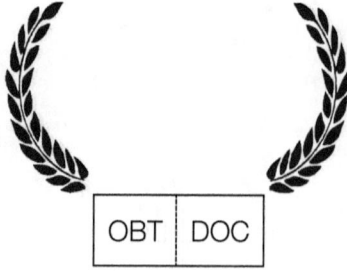

OBT	DOC

Unlimited

Obtained ITEMS AND AMOUNTS

Ritualized
INCL OBTAINED ALT PLAN

W W W W W W W W

Y Y M M D D

__ __ __ __ __ __

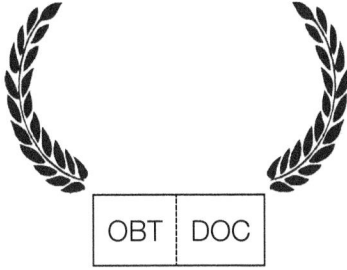

OBT | DOC

Unlimited

Obtained ITEMS AND AMOUNTS

Ritualized
INCL OBTAINED ALT PLAN

Y Y M M D D

W W W W W W W W W   __ __ __ __ __ __

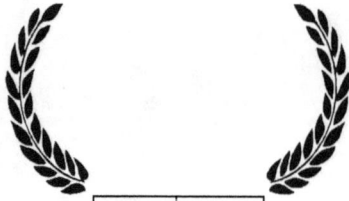

OBT	DOC

Unlimited

Obtained ITEMS AND AMOUNTS

Ritualized
INCL OBTAINED ALT PLAN

W   W   W   W   W   W   W   W

Y   Y   M   M   D   D

___ ___ ___ ___ ___ ___

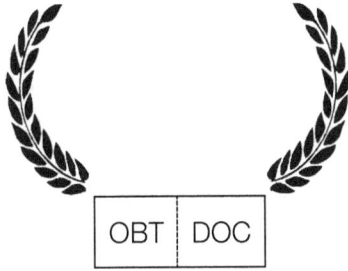

OBT | DOC

Unlimited

Obtained ITEMS AND AMOUNTS

Ritualized
INCL OBTAINED ALT PLAN

W   W   W   W   W   W   W   W

Y   Y   M   M   D   D

__ __ __ __ __ __

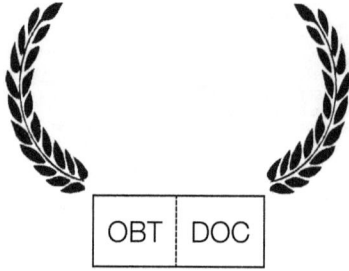

OBT | DOC

Unlimited

Obtained ITEMS AND AMOUNTS

Ritualized
INCL OBTAINED ALT PLAN

W W W W W W W W W

Y Y M M D D
__ __ __ __ __ __

© 2014 Ben G. Adams
Unboxing Press, Inc.
New York, NY

www.ingramcontent.com/pod-product-compliance
Lightning Source LLC
Chambersburg PA
CBHW060022030426
42334CB00019B/2140